SAME JOB
NEW LIFE

DANIEL BOND

DEDICATION

To my four best friends;
my beautiful family

CONTENTS

ACKNOWLEDGMENTS

Thank you to all our friends, family and colleagues who
have played their own part in this great adventure

INTRODUCTION

'The world is still young and we are all pioneers'
Anon

I live and work on the other side of the world to my employer. I have spent the last eight years living in Australia, while being employed full-time by a company in London. I do not have a unique skill set; neither am I somehow irreplaceable. I do exactly what I would do in the London office; except that I do it from my home office in our little house by the beach, on the other side of the world. I am an ordinary employee, living an extraordinary lifestyle.

Ten years ago I was one of the millions of middle-management, middle-aged people commuting into the big city. I was exhausted, bored and stressed; deeply frustrated that I didn't get to spend enough time with my young family. I was a walking stereotype.

Now, I am writing this book to that person who was me ten years ago. I know that person, my former *alter ego* or other self is still on that train because I see 'me' every time I go back. I see the exhaustion, the tension

1

and the frustration and I remember it only too well.

Only it's not me. Not anymore. That tense, tired, dispirited person isn't me; it's more likely to be you; which is why I imagine you are reading this book. It's certainly the reason why I am writing it: To give you and the other millions of exhausted, stressed, dissatisfied commuters a vision which may inspire and give them - and you - hope. I want to let as many people as possible know that there are alternatives to the daily grind in and out of the city; different and far more attractive paths that they can take.

To do that I need to show how my life has fundamentally changed for the better over these last ten years; to write about where I have been and what I have done; to recount the triumphs and disasters along a path which, though it hasn't always been easy, is a path that I will never regret taking. Everything my family and I went through has been worth it.

Today, ten years on, I enjoy the lifestyle that we always dreamed of; I am able to see my children growing up in this amazing part of the world and to share with my wife in so many more of my family's experiences. Yet, at the same time, I have been able to continue with my career in a job that I enjoy more than ever, now that I'm not spending most of my time in train delays and traffic jams or trapped in pointless meetings.

Yet, my employer has enjoyed some very real benefits from my lifestyle change. In the last eight years - approximately two thousand working days - I have only had one or two days off sick, I have never been late for work and, with no interruptions, my working hours are focused and extremely productive. Plus, as I work Australian hours, my company can provide a round-the-clock service for our clients.

For me, the facilitator in this sea change has been technology. I work remotely from my home office or, as it is otherwise known; I am a *home based worker*, a *remote worker*, a *telecommuter* or a *teleworker*. Throughout the book I will refer to the practice as 'working from home'. Now, having lived this way for a number of years I want to share my experiences; to paint a picture of what it can really be like.

This book will show you how you can harness these rapidly changing technologies to change your life while, at the same time, becoming a more efficient and valued employee. Whether you are looking to relocate and live your dream lifestyle, or are simply looking for an improved work-life balance to your existing lifestyle; this book will show you how. We will define exactly what working from home is and explore the different ways that it can bring about significant change. We will also look at identifying your own needs and establishing what type of working from home would be most suitable for you.

This mode of working is something that countless professionals from all walks of life can do and will almost certainly be doing in the future. So why not you?

In our own way my family and I have been pioneers, taking a path less travelled. The path wasn't clearly sign-posted or well-trodden and, like all great opportunities, it wasn't advertised or pre-defined. But now, with *'Same Job New Life'* you can have a guidebook to help smooth the way and avoid some of the pitfalls. The book will even show you how you may create your own opportunities, though, of course, getting started is something that you have to do yourself. As John F Kennedy said; *'Things do not happen. They are made to happen'*.

This book is intended not only as an introduction to an idea that people may not have seriously considered before, but also to demonstrate that it is entirely possible. Would you like to escape the rat race and become a 'lifestyle pioneer' of the digital age? This possibility may, or may not, be for you, but it is a viable option that I would like you and many other people to know more about, in order that everyone can make their own informed decisions. In this book I will share how my wife and I made it happen. How we made it work and, ultimately, how it can be a genuine and sustainable lifestyle choice.

As well as a guide on how you can make it happen for you, it is also the story of my family's amazing journey which I will share with you, warts and all. I hope it will inspire and serve as something of a route-map for all those brave souls who dream of having their own adventure

1. ORDINARY EMPLOYEE, EXTRAORDINARY LIFESTYLE

'Two roads diverged in a wood, and I,
I took the one less travelled by,
And that has made all the difference'
Extract from 'The Road Not Taken' by Robert Frost

My name is Daniel Bond and welcome to my story of a journey along 'the path less travelled.' I live in a quiet beachside suburb in Western Australia and (at the time of writing) have been working from home, full-time, for a UK based company for eight years. I am married to Angela, and we have three wonderful children; Florence, Alice and Michael. Our lifestyle is one of sunshine, beaches, swimming pools and palm trees. Every day I wake up and go to work, doing the same work as I would be doing in the London office. Only I'm on the other side of the world. It's the same job, but a very different life. I'm working for the same clients, I'm working off the UK server, but I'm doing it from this amazing location on the other side of the world.

So, within the confines of my laptop, not much has changed. The environment that it sits within, however, is completely different. We are a walk to the beach and our to kids' school. Our garden has palm trees, orange trees, lemon trees and a huge frangipani tree. I listen to parrots squawking as I work and often see dolphins at the beach before my working day begins. My lunch hour is often a swim at the beach, instead of a walk up the high street, past the graffiti covered walls. My commute to work is now two seconds instead of two hours and so is my journey home; giving me at least an extra four hours every day to dedicate to doing whatever I want to do (that's twenty hours a week no longer squashed in to a busy commuter train, filled with people who are just as miserable as myself).

Maybe I'm the exception but I love my job, I always did. For me, it was everything else that I didn't love: The journey to work, the soul-less universal office environment and all of the other stuff that so many of us recognise in the day to day grind of office life the world over. With all of that 'other stuff' being taken out of the equation, I now love my job more than ever.

New adventures
In the time we have been here we have explored a great deal of Australia and Asia and have shared some amazing adventures together as a family. We have; snorkelled, swam with dolphins, ridden elephants, climbed mountains, quad biked and four-wheel driven over deserted beaches, surfed, sand-boarded, been in helicopters, camped, kayaked, been white-water rafting and the list goes on. We live in an environment where outdoor activities are encouraged and accessible, and where we can literally be in the middle of nowhere within an hour's drive. Within that hour's drive we can be in remote bush-land or on deserted beaches, or alternatively we can be in a busy, vibrant, modern city.

This environment very much suits us and, it's fair to say that, we always had a good appetite for adventure. As a family, we always tried to do exciting things on holidays and at weekends. When they were very young, we spent two weeks with Florence and Alice in rustic wooden tree houses, set amongst ancient Lycian ruins in Southern Turkey, and Michael was on safari with the rest of the family in South Africa when he was only three months old. While we were never reckless, we did always try to expose our family to different 'adventures', but these were always limited to holidays and weekends. The rest of our year was all about running as fast as we could in the rat race, funding these excursions and looking forward to the next experience that we had lined up.

We are now living and raising our family in an environment that most people spend all year saving their money for, in order to spend a two week holiday there. We live in a holiday destination all year round. We are extremely lucky but, although we are rich in good fortune, we are not rich in finances. This part of the world boasts the highest population of millionaires in the whole of Australia, but we are not one of them. I am an ordinary employee, on an ordinary salary, but am lucky enough to be living an extraordinary lifestyle.

A typical working day
In the UK a typical working day for me would begin in the early morning. Angela and I would get ourselves and the kids ready for the day and have breakfast. We would then bundle everybody in to the car and she would drop me off at the train station and then, depending on the day, she would either take the kids

off to their various day-cares before setting out on her own two hour journey to work, or take the kids home and get them ready for school. I would then wait on a cold, dark train platform before squeezing my way on to a crowded commuter train in to London. Often the train would be delayed or cancelled which would mean a longer wait on the platform followed by an even tighter squash on to the next train that arrived. After changing trains and taking the second part of my journey to work, I would then walk to the office, passing the graffiti covered walls and broken glass outside the pubs from the night before. My working day would be busy but with a back drop of the constant silent and sterile atmosphere of most offices. Lunch time would be a sandwich at the desk or a stroll around the block with colleagues before finishing up my working day in the afternoon and walking back to the train station in the early evening. The journey home would be a repeat of the one from that morning (only in reverse) consisting of squeezing in to a packed train and hoping there would be no delays. I would then be picked up at the station by Angela. She would have fed the kids already and they'd be in their pyjamas, ready for bed. If my train was on time then I would get to read them a bedtime story but if it was delayed then they would probably be asleep in the back of the car when I arrived and I wouldn't see them again until the next morning, when the same events repeated themselves for yet another day.

A typical working day for me now is that I get up early and walk our dog, 'Biscuit' on the beach. It is a beautiful sandy beach and, for most of the year, the water is crystal clear. This is a great start to anybody's day.

After walking the dog I then head home, open up my home office, switch on my laptop and see what the day has in store for me. I read emails and set up whatever I need for my upcoming working day (copying files across from the server etc). I then have breakfast with the family before doing the school run. When I am back at my desk everything is prepared and I am ready to start work. The dress for my working day is generally bare-feet, shorts, T-shirt and I have 'Biscuit' lying by my feet all day as I work.

Angela does different part-time jobs and runs a couple of small businesses, so she is around some days and not others. If she is at home then we will generally take a lunch break together and will either catch up on events or maybe go for a swim. I then continue my working day and end the day by backing up all new work to the server, logging my time and sending emails. Occasionally I will have a phone conversation with one of my colleagues back in London, but generally an email is sufficient as a hand-over of my working day.

Most days, after work I will take a run or have a swim at the beach. Not only is this good exercise but it is also a good way to 'flush through' the working day. As there is no journey home for me, there is no clear distinction between work and home. This is a common situation for home based workers, whether remote-overseas employees or self-employed home business owners and it's important to have a mechanism in place to 'segment' the day. For me, putting an activity between work time and home time definitely helps with that differentiation. With work 'closed' for the day, I can then get on and enjoy my time at home.

When I am back from my run or swim then I generally spend time with the family, before we all sit down to dinner together. Wherever possible we always try to make sure that we have all meals together and use this as an opportunity to get together and talk about our busy days.

In the years that I have been working remotely I have had trips back to the UK office and I have also been involved in expanding our business in the Australasian region, so have had trips to other parts of the country for meetings and pitches. I have always enjoyed these various trips and it is good to experience the feeling of being a part of the exciting and innovative company that I work for, but it is always great to come home and put my shorts and T-shirt back on.

Work-life balance
To me, working from home is all about the opportunity to achieve a work-life balance. Yes, we've done some wonderful things since we've lived here, but it's the smaller things where the real value lies. Without my journey to and from work I have an extra four hours available to me every day. That's nearly 1000 hours per year and (if you divide that in to 12 hour days) that's an extra 83 days per year.

Within that time I have been available to go to my kid's school assemblies, help them with their homework, go to the park or play in the garden. I have built go-karts and tree-houses with them, I have started businesses with Angela, I have trained for and run marathons, I have learnt many new skills, renovated houses and now I am writing this book. These extra hours have enabled me to be there at meal-times, to read bed-time stories to my kids, to know all of their friends and to share in their lives and have a good understanding and empathy with the various things going on in their lives. I have been Michael's soccer coach for a number of years, I have always helped Florence and Alice with their weekly paper-rounds. I have helped all my kids learn to ride their bikes and I have been there to share in all of their achievements, as they accomplish new and exciting things themselves.

This lifestyle may not be for everybody but it has been a perfect solution for me in in achieving the work-life balance that I always wanted.

CHAPTER SUMMARY

What sort of working day would you like to look forward to?

What would it consist of? By breaking it down you can begin to consider what may be involved in making it a reality.

Consider your own work-life balance. Are you happy with it or are there ways in which you would like to improve upon it?

As you go through this book we will look at ways to identify your objectives and then match them with ways of working from home that may best suit your needs.

2. MOTIVATIONS FOR CHANGE

**'Insanity is doing the same thing over and over again and
expecting different results'**
Albert Einstein

What is your motivation? Why would you want to do
this? What would it mean to you and how would it
change your life? By working from home you can
potentially live anywhere in the world, living the
lifestyle of your choice. With so much choice available,
what would you choose?

Maybe your motivations are more practical and the
ability to work from home would really make a big
difference in your day to day life. Perhaps you want to
move closer to a relative who needs help? Maybe you
want the classic sea change, with a slower paced
lifestyle in a cleaner and safer environment, with better
weather. To achieve this maybe you envisage a totally
new lifestyle somewhere far away. Perhaps you yearn
for a change of lifestyle but don't want to move so far
from home; perhaps the idea of moving to the
countryside and 'down-shifting' appeals to you. Or
perhaps you want to live overseas, but want to still be
within a reasonable distance to home. For people in the
UK, Europe has so many potential opportunities for
different lifestyles and varied costs of living. Perhaps

you live in America and want to enjoy a different lifestyle. With such a vast and varied continent there is so much choice available for different lifestyles. Maybe your criteria are the opposite of many others and you live in a sleepy town and want to up the pace and experience living in the big city.

Maybe it's not location that motivates you. Perhaps you have a hobby or a passion that a change in lifestyle could benefit from? Skiing, water-skiing, scuba diving, surfing, horse riding?

My motivations
My motivations were simple; spending more time with my family and sharing new experiences together with them. I was later than many others to parenthood and when kids arrived I loved it and really saw it as a blessing. I think being a Dad is the best job in the world. I've never wanted to spend all week working and then play golf for a whole day every weekend. For me weekends have always been about spending time with my family.

I had been commuting in to London, along with thousands of others for the best part of ten years. I was caught in the rat race with a two hour train commute, each way. I was a stressed out and exhausted with too much to do and too little time. I had been blessed with a beautiful young family that I did not see anywhere near enough of. I looked around on the commuter train each day and guess what I saw? Yep, pretty much everyone else, looked just like I felt.

Slowing down, improving my lifestyle and having more

time to spend with my family was exactly what I wanted for this chapter in my life. When I was younger, there is no way that I would have wanted to do this: Miss out on the action of a busy life with the excitement of a blossoming career and the financial reward that it brings? No way. But right at that time, it was perfect - and still is.

I wanted to share in the lives of my family and really appreciate what I had. I did not want to be another statistic dissatisfied with his lot. I looked around and saw so many of my peer group trapped in the cycle of having to provide their kids with a certain lifestyle (and an endless supply of consumables) in order to atone for the fact that they have no time for them - the irony being that they have no time because they have to spend so many hours at work in order to buy all this stuff. I probably generalise too much, but that was the view from my seat on the train and I knew that I did not want it for me.

Dissatisfaction in the workplace

I knew that I wasn't the first person to feel like this and I certainly wouldn't be the last - but it was my life racing by and I wanted to do something about it. I wanted to escape the rat race, to break out of the conventions that I felt trapped in. What were these 'conventions' that I wanted to escape? Going to work and being paid: Why is this bad? To be earning money is good. So, what makes us unhappy or dissatisfied with that?

It is not easy to identify what it is that makes us dissatisfied with our work; there are probably numerous factors. A situation often occurs where we become unhappy with our current job and find a reason to attach to it: 'My boss doesn't appreciate me' or 'They don't pay me enough' or any number of other reasons. We then move to another position and are happy for a while but then after a short time this job also breeds dissatisfaction for the same or similar reasons; and so the cycle goes on. How many of us have either done this ourselves or witnessed it in others? This is a common pattern within the workplace that indicates that the dissatisfaction felt by the individual lies *within* them, and they simply *map* the cause of it on to some external thing in their working environment.

One thing I would suggest makes people unhappy about their work is how much of time they are required to dedicate to it, in proportion to how much time they have available to do other things. They feel these unbalanced ratios are forced upon them and, as a consequence, their working life may represent something of a controlled regime, which they have little control over. Generally the modern day working culture is so deeply rooted in our society that it is often difficult to fit anything else in. The demands on our time are often such that most people spend far more time at work than they do at home. The workplace, and tools that we use, have become so sterile that we feel de-humanized as we sit there staring at a screen for hours and days and years on end. The pressure to maintain this intense working lifestyle and to deliver results is such that stress levels in humans are at an all-time high. Our work-life balance is becoming increasingly off-balance.

These are obviously sweeping generalisations but, even so, I'm sure they are situations that many people would recognise. But are they new? Just because computers force us to sit in a certain way and limit the time spent talking and interacting in a traditional sense, are these new problems? Surely a computer is just a machine and haven't humans been operating machines in a mechanical way ever since the industrial revolution?

It could be said that; just as every younger generation believes they invented sex, every older generation believes that they invented dissatisfaction. Even though it is a good many years ago now, people still refer to the British TV sitcom 'The Good Life', when discussing dissatisfaction at work and the alternatives available. For those of you that are not familiar with it; the show was about a suburban husband and wife who decided to break free from the trappings of modern corporate life and live a fully sustainable life in suburbia. The situation that the husband finds himself in, and the feelings he has towards his work, are very relevant for many of us today but this was 20 or 30 years before computers were even used in the workplace. The character, Tom, designs the little plastic toys that used to be found in children's cereal boxes. It is not the work that he has come to dislike but rather than 'trap' that he sees his working life to have become. Sound familiar?

The big difference between then and now is that we have the opportunity to improve our situation. Technology is something that can potentially minimize human input, but it can also empower. This isn't a recent thing; in days gone by, a machine came along to do a job quicker which potentially minimized the human input in the process, but also freed up that person's time to spend doing other things. The most recent brand of 'technology' is digital and the changes that this has brought about are huge. We really are living in an exciting era of a 'digital revolution'. This technology drives a great many changes in working processes but the really big shifts are in communication and how people interact with each other. Ask yourself; will your personal history know you as a victim of the digital revolution or as a pioneer of it; harnessing its capabilities to enable you to explore new ways to live your life?

What have been your motivations that have led you to this point?

My immediate *'why'* was my family. Those primary, and conscious, motivations were born out of the situation that existed for me at the time - the set of circumstances that made up my everyday life. However, looking back I realise that there were other, probably subconscious, influences at work also. Things from my past that helped shape the person that I had become and probably played a role in leading me to this point.

These became apparent to me when I sat down and considered what my motivations were and what I had experienced in my life that may have brought these about. I'm sure you would also benefit from this exercise. Often your immediate motivations are simply brought about as a reaction to the current circumstances in your life. Why not dig a bit deeper and you may discover that you unearth some things that you really *do* want rather than just simply the things happening in your life right now that you *don't* want?

USA

Back in my University days, I was fortunate enough to spend each summer working in America. I had the time of my life. I was young and loved my US summers but, unfortunately, when college was done and I was in the workplace, I could no longer take four months off each year to enjoy the summer. I was stuck with English summers from now on. While I was lucky enough to have a steadily progressing career, there was still always that kid inside that yearned for the carefree days of times gone by and the sunshine. Anybody that has travelled will know that, while it is great to broaden your horizons and have new experiences, it is sometimes difficult to come back and resettle in to the 'norm.'

That summertime dude was still living inside me. In fact he still lives inside me. I would look at the other people on the commuter train and think to myself 'Lucky I'm not like them; stressed, getting old and caught up in the rat race'. However, as the years went by it was becoming crystal clear that I was actually one of those myself and that there were probably younger guys looking at me thinking; 'Lucky I'm not like him; stressed, getting old and caught up in the rat race.'

Dot com bubble

Before joining my current company, I had spent the previous four years working tirelessly towards a single goal with another company. I had joined the company early on in digital development and pretty soon we were perfectly placed at the centre of the dot com boom. We were a small, tight-knit team who were all young and enjoying those exciting times together. We worked hard and we partied hard. We all spent so much time at work that at times it felt like we all lived at the office together. The company was making plenty of money and our frequent company parties were legendary, with no expense spared. It was an exciting time and felt like it would just keep going.

In a short space of time our small company had become a huge enterprise with hundreds of people, overseas offices and plenty of acquisitions going on. The day came when we looked to 'float' the company on the London Stock Exchange and I would stand to make a good deal of money from our IPO, with the stock options that I had been offered.

Everything was rosy when suddenly, almost overnight; the dot com bubble burst and our company went down with it. Hindsight would say that we expanded too rapidly but our growth was based upon the predictions of the market we were in. Our growth trajectory was steep, as the predictions were so positive and needless to say when the bubble burst we came crashing to the ground. All employees were let go with very little to show for our time and efforts and, with no IPO, our stock options had disappeared, along with the company, leaving our hopes and dreams shattered.

However, the professional experience I'd gained over those intense few years had equipped me well and it didn't take long to get back on my feet and I have been very fortunate since. I have always worked hard for my current employer and will continue to do so, but I learnt a very important lesson with this episode from my past. It taught me about achieving a healthy work-life balance and I have seldom worked late nights or weekends since then. I have only ever *liked* a company since and will never *love* another company in the same all-consuming and unsustainable way. During that time I had no work-life balance and, just as our company had over-stretched; I had also over-stretched in my commitment. I learnt that life should be more than just work and it taught me that, although a company is a collective of individuals, your objectives and your company's objectives may not always be aligned. A company exists to generate revenue, while a human exists to live a life to the fullest potential. I learnt that a life lived only for work is a life only half lived.

Overseas secondments
At that previous company I generally managed some of our larger and more long term projects and this sometimes involved overseas trips. One of the most memorable of these was a secondment to Wellington in New Zealand. The brief overview was that there were two companies merging and we were a part of a whole host of different businesses who were deployed to 'knit' them together. We were working on their technical migration and were working alongside other technical companies that had been brought in to share the responsibility. Due to the time difference it was suggested that I relocate to New Zealand for a short time to get the project rolling.

Upon arrival I discovered that the clients (the two merging companies) were former fierce competitors and hated each other. Both sides did not want a merger and everybody was doing their best to make it as difficult as possible. On top of this I also learnt that the companies that we had been teamed up with, to work alongside, were *our* competitors. They were extremely threatened by our being involved and saw us as a precocious London company trying to break in to their space. I also discovered that my company had made promises that we were in no position to deliver and that I was the 'sacrificial lamb' who had been 'fed to the wolves' as an appeasement.

This was a very difficult and challenging experience professionally but within a few weeks I managed to achieve good working relationships with most of the people that I was involved with. We put aside the politics with the various companies involved and instead focused on working together as a team of individuals. After four months I was brought back to London, as the whole project had come to an inevitable bad end with the two merging companies deciding not to merge after all.

This experience taught me many things that are relevant to where I find myself today; I learnt about the importance of candid and concise communication when working in a different time zone. I learnt that I really liked that part of the world and the people I worked with (both Australians and New Zealanders) and most of all I learnt the importance of finding solutions, no matter how difficult and messy a situation may appear.

CHAPTER SUMMARY

Recognise that 'If you keep doing what you're doing then you'll keep getting what you're getting.'

Consider your own dissatisfaction and try and identify; what it is, what it's derived from and what it may take to cure it.

Identify your immediate motivations for change. These will generally be formed out of the things you *don't* want.

Dig deeper to explore other motivations. These may give a better indication of what you *do* want.

3. WORKING FROM HOME: IS IT FOR YOU?

'Change before you have to'
Jack Welch

Working from home is increasingly becoming an achievable lifestyle option for people from a variety of different professions around the world, but let's start looking at if it is right for you.

Could you do your job remotely?
Probably the first question to ask would be; is your job something that you could do remotely? There are potentially suitable professions that immediately spring to mind for a home based working environment, such as; a writer or foreign-correspondent, a computer programmer or web developer etc. Likewise there are others that you clearly wouldn't be able to do remotely, such as; a school teacher, a bus driver, hairdresser or a chef etc. So, is your job something that you could potentially do remotely? You'd be the best judge of that yourself, but one thing I will encourage you to do, is not write off your chances too early. You may think that your job may not be suitable as it's not immediately obvious how it would work, or that you've never heard of anybody else doing it before. Don't let that deter you. The best opportunities in life are always the ones

that you have to go looking for, or even to create yourself. The types of jobs that can be done remotely are constantly broadening with the increase of different professions working off of a computer. If your deliverables, or the service that you provide, is done on a computer then that's a good start. If that computer is hooked up to a centralized server or network, and your output is either delivered or shared via that server or network, then I would say that the signs are looking good. That, in itself is working independently and working from home is basically working independently of others and in a location away from the office.

Change: Is it for you?

How comfortable are you with change? If you are looking to 'change your life' then you must accept that this will involve some 'change.' Sounds obvious, I know, but it is something that requires emphasising. Embracing change and facing up to new challenges is a romantic image that we all like to fantasize about. We like to read about it in books and watch it in movies and picture ourselves as the hero or heroine taking on these new challenges. However, when it comes to reality, we are all different. Not all of us deal with change in the same way. We all have different comfort levels with it, and some of us struggle to embrace it or to get excited by it.

The nature of a remote worker is that of working on your own. Working alone can mean different things to different people, depending on their interpretation. I would say that a good indicator as to whether this would be right for you or not would be to ask yourself what you think working from home would mean to you.

What would be the one word or phrase that you would associate it with? It could mean; isolation, loneliness, loss of visibility, lack of recognition. Or it could mean; independence, freedom, autonomy, opportunity, a challenge. In my experience I would say that working from home can be all of these things, but if I had to choose just one word it would be 'opportunity.'

There is something very comforting about the *thought* of doing something. We happily day dream and imagine how perfect the holiday will be or what a beautiful sunny day it will be for the wedding. For many of us it is more comfortable to let things remain a daydream rather than run the risk that the reality will not live up to our expectations and our day dream will be ruined. We've all been there.

Many of us have been at countless workplace 'goodbye' presentations where somebody is leaving to go travelling, start a new job, have a baby etc. Many of us return to our work station with a mixture of feelings; some are envious of their former colleague's new challenges and some are content that they have the security of their daily routine to keep their lives ordered and unchanging.

Everyday things are happening that are changing our lives; some for the good, some not so good. It sometimes feels that we don't have the control over our lives that we used to, as change is thrust upon us at such a speed. No sooner have we just got to grips with one piece of new technology than it has been out-moded and we have to go out and buy a new one, because the old one is no longer compatible.

When we are younger most of us are actively seeking change in order to experience new challenges and possible thrills and adventures. Generally when we get older, change becomes less welcome. However, as the cliché goes; 'change is inevitable' and never more so than in today's fast paced, high technology world.

Are you up for changing your life? Honestly? Whether change excites us or scares us we need to accept it and work with it. If the thought of making a radical change in your life and taking you and your loved ones out of your known comfort zone makes you a little scared, then that doesn't necessarily mean you shouldn't do it, or that you're not the right person for the job. It simply means that you're human.

Would your personality suit it?
Research shows that 'introverts' are much better suited to work remotely than 'extroverts'. Although we tend to have stereotypical images of introverts and extroverts and tend think that these are ways of behaviour (as in, we choose to act like this), interestingly whether we are introvert or extrovert is stamped in to our DNA and will be a constant throughout our lives.

Personally I do not like the idea that I am an introvert as it conjures images of someone who is shy and awkward, but looking at the definition, I probably do match that profile. The definition of an introvert, in this context, is somebody who is focused, creative and actually works best making independent decisions without the need for peer approval.

Extroverts on the other hand need to be around other people and thrive on the interaction that it brings. They do not deal well with making decisions independently of others as they need the collaboration and the recognition that comes with it. It's interesting that, statistically, there are many extroverts who become entrepreneurs and actually struggle with the isolation and so return to an office based environment. They are attracted to the image of it (being the boss of a large company with lots of employees) but the environment that is required on the road to that large office is not anything that they enjoy (working alone and making independent decisions). What type are you?

What are your ambitions?

Are your ambitions defined by your career or are they defined by your lifestyle? One great thing about working from home is that you are potentially able to satisfy both of these. However, in my experience, while my lifestyle has vastly improved over the years, my career development has not. I enjoy my work and my role suits me perfectly but, it's fair to say, that I have not climbed any higher on the career ladder during the years that I have been working remotely. I am not complaining about this at all, and have been more than compensated in the lifestyle that I am able to enjoy, but it is an important factor in considering this as an option for you. I cannot say for a fact that all remote workers would be over-looked for promotions over their office based colleagues but I would say that it would be important to consider what potential ramifications there may be in your own career development, and how much this may concern you.

A colleague of mine started working for my present company at roughly the same time as I did. Being from different backgrounds we worked in different disciplines but collaborated often on various projects. In the years that have passed he has now risen to be joint CEO of the whole company and has got there by hard work and dedication. He is not a stereotypical 'corporate beast', achieving success by ruthlessly stepping on people. Rather, he is intelligent, hard-working and a very good people-person with excellent communication skills. There are heavy demands on his time and so he lives close to the office. This way he doesn't have to waste too much of his day travelling in to work and is able to maximise the time available to him to be able to spend with his young family. Like all of us, he is balancing his time and his responsibilities and, from what I can see, making a great job of it. He is well respected professionally, well remunerated for his hard work and has a good family life.

He and I have taken two very different paths and now have two totally different day to day experiences. These are both very unusual stories as, in a twelve year time-frame, the majority of people's career paths will typically involve a few side-ways steps with a change of employer perhaps and may be a couple of promotions along the way. It is unusual for two people to stay with one company for that long and, in that time, to have such contrasting career paths. It is, however, a true story and serves as a good illustration as to what outcomes can be possible with the different choices that we make. We both chose our paths and are both happy with our choices, based on what we wanted to achieve.

There are so many different paths available for us to take in our lives. With hindsight, some may turn out to be better choices than others but generally we make the decisions that we believe to be right for us at the time. Most times we'll never know what the other path would have been like and we simply make the best of the one that we have chosen.

I chose the path less travelled for reasons that I believe were right for me at the time. I have already described my motivations and some of the things that helped shaped my life to the point of making that decision. My ambitions were less defined by my career at that point and more defined by my personal life. It was right for me and I will never regret it. However, that is not to say that it is right for everybody.

What are your expectations?
A very important part of making this lifestyle change successful is to get your expectations in the right place. Like goals, if expectations are too high then they no longer serve as something to aim for, but rather a stick to beat yourself with.

We have brought our family to a whole new environment and we are very happy – but it is not perfect. Where we live is not perfect. My working arrangement is not perfect. There will always be things that we miss about the environment that we used to live and work in. One of my children brought a drawing of 'their perfect holiday' home from school and it was of a snowy landscape. We smiled as she told us that most of the people in her class had drawn something similar. Where we had come from in the UK 'the perfect holiday' drawing would almost certainly be sunshine and beaches.

I'm sure you'd agree that understanding that nothing is perfect is common sense. However, when it comes to a life change, the unrealistic and futile pursuit of perfection becomes apparent in most of us. We are all looking for something 'better' and it takes a while to get a handle of what level of 'better' we can realistically expect.

Accepting that your new experience will be made up of both good and bad things is part of the adventure. You ride the good and bad together and grow stronger from it, with the highs being fully appreciated as a result of experiencing the lows. Expecting perfection is a fast track to disappointment and a 'boomerang' back to where ever it is that you came from. Be aware of the pursuit of perfection. In my own experience, it doesn't exist and can only lead to disappointment.

CHAPTER SUMMARY

Identify your own comfort level with change.

Clearly define your expectations from this lifestyle change. Are your goals achievable?

Ask yourself; would working from home suit you?

What are your career ambitions and how compromised would they be by taking on a working from home role?

4. DIFFERENT TYPES OF WORKING FROM HOME

'Change is the only constant.
Hanging on is the only sin'
Denise McCluggage

Let's now look at the different types of working from home and start to consider how these can translate in to meaningful changes in your life. The different types of working from home have been split into five categories, based on 'degrees of remoteness.' They have been categorized in this way in order that we can explore them and try to best match them to your own needs. This is by no means a definitive list but it is a good guide as to what possibilities are available for you to consider. In each one we look at lifestyle scenarios that these may potentially include.

Category 1: Working from home.
Changing your working arrangement so that instead of being office based, you are home based, with the option of going in to the office if required.

This is clearly the option with the least amount of change required and may not result in any radical lifestyle changes. However, you would potentially have more time available without having to travel in to the office. This category would suit somebody who's personal needs may have possibly changed in their life but who still has a requirement to continue working, either for income purposes or career development. Perhaps a new baby has come along and you as parents are feeling stretched with the demands that this brings. Looking after a baby or young child is not possible in addition to carrying out your full-time duties, but the proximity to a child-care facility or family member who could look after the child may be of huge benefit. This category would suit parents of a young family for the same reasons. Being there to take your kids to school means an awful lot and your work can potentially start earlier or finish later in order to fulfil both your duties as a parent and as an employee. Perhaps a family member has become ill and being home based would mean greater availability for caring for them and more peace of mind that you have closer proximity if required. This may also be a good option for somebody who is actually very happy with their home life and would simply like to spend more time there than just weekends. Perhaps you have a hobby that you are only really able to do at weekends but, without the commute in to the office, you are now able to enjoy after work each night also. You may be successfully working from home already to some extent (doing a day from home once in a while) and can now see how you could potentially expand on this and transition yourself to a full-time work from home situation.

Category 2: Moving to a new home.
Your new home might be a little further away from the office so working from home is your primary role but you can still get in to the office on occasion if required.

Maybe you could afford a bigger house by moving to a new area and so this motivation prompted the move and working from home made it possible. Perhaps you've relocated to an area that is best for a specific hobby or interest of yours such as ocean based pastimes like sailing or surfing. Maybe, you've just started a family and want to move closer to your own parents for that all important support network, and involve them in the life of your new family. Perhaps you're in a relationship with somebody that lives in a different area and working from home makes it possible to relocate and work from there. Maybe when you left college you came to the big city for the excitement of a young single life and now you've started a family and want to move back to the area where you are originally from.

Category 3: Moving to a remote location within the same country.

You relocate to a totally different part of the country and can explore a new and exciting lifestyle. You are a full-time remote worker who cannot get in to the office.

The previous two categories both suit scenarios that are practically orientated. This one and the following two are more lifestyle change orientated. Depending on where you live in the world there is generally a good scope for exploring different lifestyles within the boundaries of the same country. If you live in the UK for example then a move in this category could potentially mean moving to the Scottish Highlands for its spectacular and dramatic landscape. It could include relocating to the Cotswolds region for the picturesque villages and laid back lifestyle. Maybe you have an interest that is specific to a region such as mountain climbing and you want to bring about a lifestyle change that places you right in the heart of this activity. If you live in other countries there are similar scenarios that would apply to the different regions that you would be more familiar with than I; such as in the USA where a more laid back lifestyle is potentially available in New England or the Carolinas. A warmer climate can be found in Florida and California, and skiing and mountain climbing are obviously specific to mountainous regions. Huge varieties of different lifestyles are often available within the same country and working from home makes these lifestyle changes possible.

Category 4: Moving overseas, but to a location that doesn't require a visa.

You relocate overseas and can explore a totally new lifestyle without having to obtain work permits or visas. You are a full-time remote worker who cannot get to the office.

Obviously large countries such as Canada and the USA are expansive enough to be able to offer hugely varying lifestyles within the same country. Australia is the only country which is also a continent and very different lifestyles are available there too, within the same nation. But people who live in smaller countries often feel that a significant lifestyle change will require moving overseas. Living in a different country, without having to obtain new visas or passports, is possible today for many people who are fortunate enough to be able to move freely between national boundaries and work in different countries. This category has commonly suited people from European Union countries who are able to live and work in any member nation. So, people from the Germany could potentially relocate to France, Spain, Italy or many other different European countries that offer varied and exciting lifestyle changes. Many UK residents have been living throughout the EU on this basis but, post-Brexit, this is likely to change or at least become more difficult to achieve.

Obviously with the potential for a more radical lifestyle change comes an increased amount of factors for consideration such as; different languages, different customs, different currency and so many more. Using Europe as an example; the different countries may be geographically close together but they are widely separated by their histories, culture, attitudes and lifestyle.

This option would also be suitable for the many professionals that have dual nationality. Maybe your parents are migrants and you are curious to go and experience 'the old country' for yourself. You've heard so much about it and feel that it is somewhere that is a part of who you are, but you have experienced very little of it yourself. There may be friends and family that would love to have you come and share in their lives and experience their lifestyle. Working from home makes this a real possibility.

Category 5: Moving far overseas to a location that will require new visas or emigration
You relocate far overseas and are emerged in a totally new and exciting lifestyle. You will need to obtain work permits or visas and you are definitely a full-time remote worker who cannot get in to the office.

This option is probably the best one for people who are looking to making a very significant change in their lifestyle. However it is also the one that is potentially the most challenging, both from a planning perspective and from an implementation perspective. Part of the planning will likely require lengthy and complicated visa applications etc, which you will have to try and navigate your way through. When you are working remotely from your new location on a day to day basis it is likely you will be working on a totally different time-zone and are more likely to experience the feeling of isolation in your professional life. These are just a couple of examples of how this option can be potentially challenging.

This may suit people that already have a destination in mind and working from home presents itself as a great opportunity to make it happen. Perhaps you visited somewhere on a holiday or while back-packing and really like the idea of spending some time living there. Perhaps you are already decided on a temporary relocation or are possibly planning to emigrate. Working from home could be an option that you may not have seriously considered before and, now you have been introduced to the idea, you can really see how this could help facilitate your move. Perhaps you have been working remotely for a while; you are now feeling comfortable with this mode of work and can see how you could transfer this lifestyle to an overseas location.

Matching your needs
Depending on your individual set of circumstances, you may read through the five categories and may or may

not know which one would best suit your needs. But don't worry; the next chapter is all about working to identify what your objectives are. Once you have clearly identified your objectives then you may wish to revisit the categories to see which option is a right fit for you.

Remember they are only a guide and it may be best to combine them in order to create a solution that is workable for you. For example, it may be that you really want to move to the other side of the world and live your dream lifestyle (category five) but after exploring the reality of it you realise that you are not ready for this yet. So you decide to spend a year doing category one (working from home) in order to see how you manage with working from home and also to use that time to apply for the necessary visas that you'll require. Alternatively it may be that you get started on making a category five lifestyle change but discover that you are not able to meet the visa requirements. Having done your due diligence and being mentally prepared for a move overseas, you then switch to a category four instead. Similarly you could be a remote worker on the other side of the world (category five) for a time, but miss home or are just ready for a new challenge. You could therefore swap working from home from your overseas location for working from home within the same country as your employer (category three).

Another alternative may be that you really like the idea of having your own adventure but are not planning a permanent move right now. In which case, you can do any of these working from home types on a temporary basis, with a view to going to back to being office based within a given time-frame. For example, perhaps you have just started a family and your child is pre-school age. You know that once your child starts school that your maneuverability will be more limited and your holidays will be fixed to the school holiday calendar. You want an adventure before this inevitable phase kicks in and so you and your family spend six months living and working from home in Tuscany or Florida or Australia or anywhere that you've dreamed of. After six months your life and career can resume as before but the priceless experience of those six months will be with you and your family for the rest of your lives.

This temporary period of working from home could equally be a way of 'testing the waters' for a future permanent move. For example, you may like the idea of moving to the other side of the world but are concerned you may get too home sick and miss family and friends too much. You could potentially spend a few months working remotely from that location to experience it first. If you like it; great, you can make a start on applying for the relevant visas etc for a future move. If not; fine, now you've got it out of your system and you can happily get on with your life - happier and more contented with things as they are.

These are just a few possible scenarios, but there are many occasions in your life when you may want to take some time to experience something different, or just change priorities. Working from home makes this possible.

CHAPTER SUMMARY

There are many different ways that working from home can be used to make a big difference to your life.

Match your objectives with the type of working from home that best suits needs.

You can also combine these types together in order to match your needs. For example start with one and move to another.

None of these have to be permanent. They can be done on a temporary basis either for a fixed time-frame, or as test-case for a future permanent move.

DANIEL BOND

5. IDENTIFYING YOUR OBJECTIVES

'If you can dream it, you can do it'
Walt Disney

So, you've looked at your motivations; the reasons behind your desire to bring about change. You've now looked at some of the options available to you in working from home. Now let's start to look at your objectives. Your objectives are the things that you wish to achieve in this change that you are looking to make.

Our main objectives were that we wanted to have a better lifestyle and we wanted more time with our family, but how could we achieve that? What did it mean in reality? What did this 'lifestyle' consist of? What components would it take to construct this dream that we had? We began to put together a wish-list. On this list we wanted; more time, better weather, a slower pace of life, an outdoor life, opportunities for our whole family to do new and exciting things that were not currently available to us, experience new places, good education, good sporting facilities, good career opportunities, to live somewhere with a 'holiday feel' but with a modern infrastructure, I wanted to fly aeroplanes, Angela wanted to wind-surf, we wanted to be near the ocean and so our list went on. We looked at our list and viewed potential locations accordingly.

Create a wish-list

What would be on your wish-list? What does your dream lifestyle look like? If you can picture that life clearly enough then you're one step closer to making it happen. I don't mean the 'think it and it'll happen' coffee-table psychology. I mean that if you create a strong enough vision of something in your mind, you can then start drawing up a clear plan for how you can bring this about. Look at it as if it were your dream home that you were building; if you knew exactly what it looked like in your mind, then you can draw up clear and concise blue-prints that would make actually building the house so much easier and more achievable. Alternatively, if you only have a few vague ideas of a house and draw up a number of different sets of plans (all equally vague), then that house is never likely to be your dream home, if it ever gets built at all. It's the same process as building a dream and, the first stage of making your dream life a reality is creating your vision.

Day dream

In starting to create your vision I would definitely recommend that you deploy some 'blue-sky thinking'. Really use your imagination to begin to paint a picture of what your dream lifestyle looks like, without limits. Daydream. Find a daydream that makes you feel good and go with it. It may be something that you haven't thought of in years but it comes back to you, or it may be something that you think about every day on the way into work. It's not just about a location but piecing together the vision of a whole lifestyle. What is really important to you and what is it that you will need to do in order to achieve these things?

Do not cloud your vision too early with worries about 'how am I going to manage that'. Start crafting your vision by focusing on the end result and then you can work back from there. By all means, create as far reaching a vision as you like, but make sure that it is true to you and your personality. For example it may be that you look at our five different types of working from home and be drawn to level five. You envisage a totally new lifestyle, far away from your existing one. However, a move like this would most likely involve the most planning and most uncertainty. If you know that you do not deal well in uncertain situations then it may be that; you may spend time on a beautiful beach - but that time would be spent worrying about all of the risks that it has taken to get there. Ask yourself; what is your comfort level on the risk versus reward ratio? Is this vision really achievable for you, or does it require going so far out of your comfort zone that you know the pain will outweigh the gain? Some people can mentally compartmentalise thoughts on risk and put them in to a context that doesn't interfere with other areas of their lives, while others cannot sleep at night with the constant fear of the worst case scenario playing out. We are all programmed differently. Your daydream should make you feel good. If your daydream is causing you to experience discomfort then it may be worth trying to identify what is causing it.

Focus on what you want and not what you don't want
An important thing in identifying your objectives is to focus on what you *do* want, rather than what you *don't* want. As we have said, the way to define this dream lifestyle is to construct it in your mind first, and the key point here is that it will be made up of the things you do

want, not the things you don't want. The things you don't want will help in the early stages of the elimination process, but they do not feature in the makeup of what you do want. It is no good sitting spewing vitriol about the awful weather and terrible train system, this is simply going to fill you with negative emotion and make you feel bad.

Often, when we consider making big changes to our lives we generally do it as a reaction to the things that we don't want. We want to reject our current situation and escape to a better one. This carries with it a lot of strong emotions and we often believe that we want a total clear out of everything; to run away and start again from scratch. It doesn't always have to be this way and when you sit down and look at things unemotionally you'll probably find that there are a lot of things that are good in your life and other areas that can be fixed with a bit of work. You don't need to 'throw the baby out with the bathwater' and, luckily for us today, we don't have to.

In the past, relocating, especially somewhere as far as Australia, often meant giving up everything and everyone you've ever known and saying goodbye to it forever. Nowadays it doesn't have to be like that. With travel, communications and technology we all live and operate on a global scale, even if it's simply watching live sport from another country on the TV. Why not do an audit of all the things in your life, reject the bad and look at ways of retaining or improving the good?

Avoid the stereotypes
I don't know what your dream life is, but one thing I do know is that it won't be the same as mine or anybody else's. It will be unique to you. We are unique individuals, we all like doing different things and we all have different tastes. One thing I would advise at this stage is that you try and avoid the stereo-types. It may have been a long time since you really allowed yourself to think about a 'dream come true', may be not even since childhood for some of us. In the absence of a clear and easy answer to the question 'what do I really want' we may feel compelled to go with the obvious.

There is a default dream life that we've been fed by the media over the years. It features sandy beaches, palm trees, red sports cars, big houses, golf courses and so on. We all know the one. Try to avoid being influenced by these images and by other such stereotypes. You may not like the beach or have no interest in golf. You may like the countryside and hills and trees instead, not everybody likes hot weather. The likes and preferences that are unique to you may be buried fairly deeply in your mind, but they are in there somewhere; we all have things that make us happy. Use some of that 'blue sky thinking' that we mentioned earlier and really dig down and retrieve them from wherever they're buried.

Create a vision together
It is essential to consider the impact on personal relationships with regard to your potential relocation. When you are identifying your objectives, make sure that you do this together with whoever will be involved in this change in lifestyle. It's no good making a list of everything that you want and assuming everybody else

will want it too, or trying to force these wishes upon others. This change will involve everybody and will require a team effort. If you do not share the same objectives then you will really struggle to make this a long-term sustainable move.

The other important thing that I feel the need to mention is that; if your objectives are for a relocation as an attempt to solve relationship problems then you may be disappointed. If you and your family are not seeing enough of each other and a change of lifestyle would mean you spent more time together then that's great. However, if you and a partner are experiencing problems in your relationship, then it's very unlikely that relocation would solve this. This is probably a similar logic that couples use when they decide to have a baby together; because they are experiencing relationship problems. If anything, relocation is likely to put increased strain on your relationships and, if there are any cracks then they will only become bigger with that increased pressure.

Believe in your vision
Once you have created a clear idea of what you want to achieve then stick with it. Believe in your vision and have faith in your ability to bring it about. Visualize it and see it happening in your mind. After all, if you don't believe in it and have faith in it yourself then how can you possibly convince others to believe in both your vision and your ability to make it a success?

In the early stages, when you are first contemplating the idea, there will plenty of things that have the potential to dent your belief in it. Our belief systems are fine with things that we understand and have experienced already but these belief systems do not work so well with new concepts and ideas. Also, the attitude of our friends and family can potentially de-rail us when they tell that this is a crazy idea and give us a list of reasons why it won't work: 'Somebody else could do but not you. Your job is not suitable. Your boss would never allow it', or any number of other reasons. These seeds of doubt can take a hold and stop you from developing your vision any further. It is much easier to think like that and, avoiding taking any risks keeps us safe from the fear of the unknown and of potential failure.

You need to try and put these inevitable responses in to perspective and understand why they are being said. It's not that people who respond like this are bad (they probably care about you very much and do not want to see you hurt or disappointed), but these are common human responses to unfamiliar things. Obviously you need a good sense of reality about your plans and, while you don't want to cave in to these doubts, equally it's of no benefit to simply surround yourself with people who will only tell you what you want to hear. However, there is a difference between objective reality and negative sensationalism.

When you have created a clear vision of your dream lifestyle you can then begin to research the plausibility and to draw up the blue-prints of how to go about turning this dream in to a reality.

CHAPTER SUMMARY

Ask yourself what your objectives are and which category would best suit your needs.

Put together your own 'wish-list' and try and avoid the stereotypes.

Focus on what you want, rather than what you don't want.

Don't be afraid to daydream and believe in your vision.

6. PLANNING

'It wasn't a miracle, we just decided to go'
Jim Lovell, Apollo astronaut

I love the quote at the top of the page from the Apollo 13 Commander, Jim Lovell. In this quote he is referring to the first moon landing and the fact that, it was made possible by man's actions. It started with an idea; an intention; a dream. But the reality was brought about by application, determination, testing and planning. Generally a great idea will be born from our imagination and sparked by some romantic or idealistic image, but it is not our imagination that brings it to fruition. The other part of the brain is required to move it from an idea, in to a plan, and then in to reality.

How much planning should you do?
'If you fail to plan, then you plan to fail' they say. But how much planning should you do? Your degree of planning will largely depend on the type of person you are and the level of change you are looking to make. If you are simply switching from being office based to being home based then the planning required will be limited to the logistics of the individual set of

circumstances in your personal life. If, on the other hand you are looking to relocate then that will require a totally different degree of planning.

In my own experience; I have known people who moved to Australia, having never even been there before, and loved the whole thrill of it. We have also known people who spent over five years planning every detail of their proposed move and actually gave up their jobs in order to dedicate themselves to the task on a full-time basis. We were probably somewhere between the two of these, where we wanted to feel like it was an adventure, but confident that it was an achievable and sustainable one.

Timing:

There are number of different things to consider with regards to timing. First; when is the time right for you to start to make changes in your life? I would say that there's never a perfect time to make radical changes in your life but we do them anyway and make everything fit around it. For example, if we all waited for the 'perfect time' to have children then probably none of us ever would. Most of us generally know when we are ready for change. That's why people on house renovation shows on TV are often a certain age; why men buying Harley Davidsons are often a certain age and why women starting art classes are often a certain age. I know these are generalisations but my point is that different things appeal to us when we are in a certain place in our lives; we feel it within ourselves. Mother Nature generally lets us know when we're ready, and after ten years on the commuter train and a young family that I wanted to spend more time with,

Mother Nature was positively yelling in my ear.

A good indication that you're ready is that you're reading this book right now. We generally seek out what we are looking for and, just as a mother can identify her child's cry amongst the throng of hundreds of kids, our consciousness homes in on exactly what it is that we are subconsciously looking for.

The second part of timing is to ask yourself; when you want these changes in place by? Do you have any significant milestones or deadlines that you want to be working to? For us; the window of time that we were actually working to was when our eldest daughter Florence left primary school and moved to senior school. In the UK this happens at age eleven and is a big move in a child's life. They are going from being the biggest kids in the school to being the smallest. Everything is new, and generally bigger, and they have to make new friends and in many ways their school life and their identity starts again. We didn't want Florence to have to go through all of these changes and then uproot her soon after to go through it all again somewhere else. We wanted our move to coincide with her inevitable upcoming move to a new school; in order to minimize the disruption in her personal life and her school life.

The third part of timing is in constructing a workable time-line that will enable these changes to be implemented in the best way possible. This is almost a project management task and will vary in complexity according to the level of changes you are looking to make. For example; If you are looking at relocating to another country that requires you obtaining a residency visa, then you will need to have a rough idea of how long that application process will take in order that you can factor it in to the time-line. This will avoid you walking in to your boss's office and telling them your great idea to relocate to Canada and start working from home in a week's time; and then subsequently discovering that it may take two years to obtain a residency visa.

Personal relationships

An important thing to factor in to your planning is to consider all of your personal relationships. These are intangibles that can easily be overlooked but often have a major significance in your ability to make working from home a long-term and sustainable life change. Considerations regarding your personal relationships will be unique to you, but may include; aging parents who may possibly need some degree of care, kids missing out on a support network of an extended family, close bonds with siblings or perhaps you have a situation with ex-spouses or are a 'blended' family.

Different languages

A very appealing relocation option for people in the UK is mainland Europe. In our relocation categories this is a category four and benefits from an overseas move but without having to obtain different visas or residency permits. Probably the biggest potential problem with this option however is that they will speak a different language and that is obviously a very important factor to consider in your planning.

The language barrier can not only cause difficulties from

a practical perspective but it can make you feel isolated and cut off from the larger community. Does the region of your choice speak your language and if not are you willing and capable of learning another language to a proficient level? How will you achieve this and how long will it take?

Location

Looking back to our relocation categories we see that they increase in complexity as they go, with the fifth category being the most demanding in what will be required to bring it about. If you are looking at this type of relocation then the first thing you need to do is to establish if you can indeed actually live there at all. It is not possible to gain residency status for some countries, and for those where it may be possible for you, there may be things that disqualify you such as a criminal record. Once you have established that you can live there, you then need to find out how you can live there and what the process will involve.

With our objectives in mind we identified Australia as being a place we would like to relocate to. Australia has long been a common migration path for people from the UK and, with Australia being a former British colony, there are many reminders of Australia's colonial history. In the past it was easier for British people to obtain residency in Australia and, as recently as 1960s, they wanted people so badly that they encouraged mass migration and all they asked was for a £10 contribution towards their boat journey to the other side of the world - these were known as 'Ten Pound Poms'. Those days are now gone and Australia is an independent nation that no longer offers British Citizens any special immigration privileges and all applications for residency are assessed in the same way, regardless of where the applicant has come from.

It is certainly not easy to obtain residency (and the criteria seems to be becoming increasingly harder) and every application is assessed using a 'points system' that rates you based on certain criteria, such as; whether or not your profession is on their current list of job requirements, if you have children, if you have an Australian citizen sponsoring your application and so on. It is essentially like applying for a new job with a company; they have an opening for a position and will consider people who meet the relevant criteria, and will make their decision through an application process. This is a complicated and lengthy process and, as mentioned earlier, the application processing time is something that needs factoring in to your time-line, also the rules are constantly being updated so there is no guarantee that your application will be successful.

For our own application we engaged the services of an 'emigration agency' that helped to guide our application through the complicated process. Our application was based on part professional; with my profession being on their list of requirements, and part sponsorship; as I was fortunate enough to be sponsored by my Australian relatives. Even with using an agency, our application still took a few years to process.

Luckily at the end of it all we were successful and a formal offer of 'Permanent residency' was made, with a five year time limit with which to take it up. If we did not relocate and assume residency within that time period then the offer would expire.

After living there for two years with our Permanent resident status, we would then be able to apply for Australian citizenship (this has now changed from two years to four years). Fortunately, upon gaining our citizenship we would not have to relinquish our British citizenship, as the UK and Australia have an agreement where you can have dual-nationality and hold both passports, without having to give up one or the other. This is a very fortunate thing for us as, people from many other countries are asked to relinquish their previous citizenship when they become Australian citizens. We had the opportunity to hold two passports for the rest of our lives. Had this not have been an option then I'm not at all sure we would have chosen Australia, as we probably wouldn't have wanted to give up our British citizenship. This is an important consideration for anybody relocating and especially those who are looking at working from home; if you are having to be committed on a *permanent* basis to your new location then it changes the nature of what you are looking to achieve with working from home.

Logistics in day to day living

Again this will vary according to the level of change you are proposing but it will include things such as; tax systems, schools, healthcare, exchange rates, cost of living and so on.

Another benefit that we discovered existed between the UK and Australia was in their tax system. I would be able to have my salary paid to me by my UK based company, but not pay my income tax to the UK government but to the Australian government instead; as that is where I would be domicile. Again, the tax systems are a very important thing to research in a proposed overseas relocation for working from home.

When we looked at the differences in the school system we discovered that it was actually very different to what we were used to. In the UK there is a gulf between a private school and public school. Our kids had always gone to the free public school and the standard was good, and was reasonably well funded by the government. In Australia there is also a private and public system in place but the differences and costs between them is not so large. The public schools that were available seemed to be not funded as well by the government and the results were quite a long way short of what our kids were getting for free in a public school in the UK. When we looked at private schooling, we discovered that the fees were much more reasonable than the UK (as the Australian government subsidises each child) and that the results were more comparable with our experience of the UK. On this evidence we decided that we would need to send our kids to private school in order to maintain the level of education that they were currently getting. This cost would need factoring in to our budget and, although we would prefer to get free education, we felt that we didn't want our kids' education to suffer as a consequence of this move. I should state here that this is not always the case across the whole country. There are excellent free schools around the country as well. Like anywhere, all school's results vary between areas and we were comparing the results in the particular catchment where we wanted to live with the results of the UK school that the kids were currently attending.

We found the same to be true of health care. In the UK we had free government funded healthcare and discovered that we would need to invest in private healthcare in Australia; where the basic level would cover part dental, optical and ambulance cover. This was something that we had not considered at all and was another cost that we would have to factor in. However, on the whole we learnt that most things were cheaper in Australia (at that time) and so, with a cheaper cost of living and the savings that we had, we could afford to earn less.

As well as working out a plan of action on my job, we had to consider what we should do about Angela's business. She would have to discuss the situation with her business partner and they would have to decide a way forward together.

The list was seemingly endless, with everything including exchange rates, removal costs, technology requirements, utilities, tax, and different insurances and so on. These are all important things that you will need to research if you are proposing an overseas location.

CHAPTER SUMMARY

The level of planning required will vary depending on the type of person you are and the level of change you are looking to make.

Be sensible and realistic on your timings. For example; if you are planning on making a move that requires lengthy visa applications then begin that process first.

Your planning will need to be focused on practicalities but also make sure that you include emotional considerations as well, such as personal relationships.

Relocation overseas will generally be a far more complex challenge and involve a great deal more planning.

7. SEE FOR YOURSELF

'Nothing ever becomes real till it is experienced'
John Keats

Working remotely enables you to potentially live and work anywhere in the world. But where do you want to live? It may be that you've always dreamed of living in a particular place and this book is exactly the guide you've been waiting for to make that happen. Or it may be that you like the idea of down-shifting or a change in lifestyle but are not entirely sure of what that may consist of, and what geographical location will provide the lifestyle you've been dreaming of.

Having been through the identification process in this book you will hopefully have defined the sort of relocation that would best suit your needs. On paper it looks great; but what does it look like in reality? Personally, I would recommend going to visit your potential location before committing to relocate there. Some may disagree and say it'll spoil the magic and you should just roll with it. If it were a holiday then I would agree but, as it somewhere you are looking to live then I would definitely advise having a look first. Otherwise it's a little like buying a house on the Internet, based solely on the pictures shown, and the discovering when you move in that it backs on to a busy road or is in a terrible neighbourhood. You have to view the context in order to see the whole picture.

I would advise being sensible on the timing of your trip and only make this investment when a particular location has become a place of serious consideration. For example, if you've only just begun a long residency application then I would say that a trip such as this is not yet relevant and would not be time or money well spent at this point.

Our 'look-see'

Before committing to the area where we would relocate, we went on a three week trip to our three preferred destinations in Australia. This short-list of areas was based on our experiences on holidays and a brief time that I had spent working there some years ago. This was quite an expensive holiday for a family of five, but it proved to be well worth the investment.

First, we went to a city on the East Coast where I had briefly worked previously. This was great and was definitely the most sensible location in terms of my career. The prospect of working from home meant that proximity to a major city was not of paramount importance, but not knowing how long the working from home would last, it would be wise to consider an area that would make the continuation of my career easier. However, we decided against this location as it didn't offer the degree of lifestyle change that we were seeking. Our move was primarily motivated by the dream of a better lifestyle and we didn't want to compromise at this late stage. If we were going to be moving this far then we wanted it to *feel* different.

The second place was also on the East Coast and was a good practical option, as Angela and I both had family living there who we got on with very well. My family had helped with our gaining residency and were really excited about the prospect of our living near them. This location scored better on the lifestyle change, while still having reasonably close proximity to a major city too. This was a very tough decision, as we would love to have been close to our families, but ultimately we decided that the area wasn't for us. Although we felt really guilty about it, we decided against it as we wanted this new adventure to be all ours. We wanted to meet new people and discover new places, but we knew if we lived close to our families, then our friends would be their friends and the places we went to would be places that we had had recommended to us. This is not anybody's fault but something that would happen quite naturally. If we had friends or family move near us then it would be just as natural for us to integrate them in to our lives and to comment on places that we have been to before but they have not yet visited. We wanted to feel that we were discovering new things ourselves and, although our families were understandably disappointed, they have always respected our decision and understood our reasons. They used to tell us great stories of their settling in this great country and our own decision came from an admiration of them and their tales, and a desire to emulate them. Now when we see them we have our own great stories to share with them and, I like to think that they respect us all the more for them.

The third place was on the West Coast and was the least sensible option on all counts - but it felt much more like the lifestyle that we wanted. It was the 'wild-card' and was somewhere that I had visited many years ago. Angela had never been there and I always told her how great it was and I wanted to go back to see if it was as good as I remembered. During our time in the first two locations it poured with rain constantly. We barely saw that famous Aussie sunshine at all. I told Angela not to worry as the weather on the West Coast was fantastic and the bad weather we had experienced so far would make the beautiful West Coast sunshine seem even better. When we arrived at the airport it was pouring with rain there too, and didn't stop for days.

We were becoming increasingly concerned that we had come this far with our plans and now here we were visiting our 'dream' destination and it didn't feel anything like the start of the dream lifestyle that we were hoping for. Our offer of a visa would be expiring soon and we had to 'use it or lose it'. Life back home was good. I had a good career, Angela had a good business, our kids were happy and healthy and we had a nice home and great holidays. Despite the rainy weather, the kids absolutely loved our time in Australia and were so excited when we told them that we could live there. This made it even harder because Angela and I were increasingly unsure. While we knew how demanding life could be in the rat race, it was providing a good income and a nice life for our loved ones.

The sun did eventually come out and we met some

people that we had been introduced to us by a 'friend of a friend'. We were initially reluctant to get in touch with these people, as we didn't know them at all and felt awkward about it - it was outside of our comfort zone. We'll always be glad we did, as they were to become our best friends and over the years since have always been a great support to us. They have a daughter who was the same age as our middle child Alice. These two absolutely hit it off straight away and are still the best of friends today. In getting to know a few people, we had got 'under the skin' of life in the area a bit more. We visited their daughter's school and it was exactly the sort of school that we had imagined our own kids to going to. There were things that we experienced that made us feel happier, but we were still far from convinced that this was the 'dream lifestyle' that we had been working towards for so long. We eventually decided to give it a go for two years. In this time, we would have obtained our dual nationality and then we'd see what we wanted to do from there.

Looking back, I would say that it was a blessing that in all three locations we experienced such awful weather, and by the end of our trip we were really not sure that we wanted to come at all. One of the big components to 'the dream lifestyle' is the weather. In hindsight, having bad weather allowed us to view the places more objectively and the thing that made up our minds once and for all was that we never wanted to say 'what if'. We had the opportunity; the door was open for us. If we closed it, then it would never open again and we would always be wondering what would have happened. We decided to go for it anyway and never say 'what if'. Those rainy days on holiday in Australia did not make the decision easy, but they did help to ensure that it was a decision made for the right reasons.

CHAPTER SUMMARY

Visiting your potential location, at a relevant time, is a very worthwhile investment of your time and money.

Remember to view it as somewhere to live, not somewhere to spend a holiday.

Be clear on your objectives for the move and make your decisions based on these.

Follow up on the 'friend of a friend' introductions. You never know where they will lead and are the start of having to do things that are outside of your current comfort zone.

Experiencing bad weather may be a positive thing in encouraging objective decision making and avoiding knee-jerk emotional responses.

8. MAKING IT HAPPEN

'The most effective way to do it, is to do it'
Amelia Earhart

Here is where it starts or finishes. Let's make one thing absolutely clear; whether you have the opportunity to work remotely or not will ultimately be decided by your boss. That's why it is so important that you do a good job in convincing them of the benefits. Whatever your line of work, you now need to discover and cultivate the 'inner salesperson' in order to make this happen. 'Oh no... sales?', I hear you cry. 'I thought this book was all about leaving that behind and escaping to the beach?' Sorry, not yet. You've got some serious work to do before that.

You are looking to create a need, where there wasn't one before. Your boss is quite happy with you working in the office and has no need to change that. It's up to you to create that need and to convince him of the potential benefits. If you say to your boss, 'I want you to let me work remotely.' They say 'Why should I?' You say, 'Because it would be a nice thing for you to do.' Your chance of getting what you want is not great. You have not told your boss why they should do it and what is in it for them. You have not established the need.

Establishing a need is commonplace with anything new; and this is new. It's a new way of working. Whenever a new product line comes on to the market it has to do the same. It has to create a need, where a need doesn't currently exist. Nobody was out there looking to buy a Smart Phone ten years ago; they had not been invented, and yet today it seems that we can't live without them. We all *need* one. Creating a need is something that entrepreneurs and marketers are well versed in, but we're not all entrepreneurs and marketers. So, how does the average person achieve this?

If this all seems a bit daunting and new, then let's look at it in a familiar way that we can all understand; let's look at it from an employment perspective. You do not simply decide on a job you want and walk in to the company and tell them that's what you want and so could they please set up a desk for you to start working there. You decide on what sort of a job you want and then apply to a business that has a job like that available. Whether you get that job or not is ultimately the company's decision; but that decision will be made based on you, and how well you convince them that you are the right person for that job. If you say to your potential boss, 'I want you to let me work here.' They say 'Why should I?' You say, 'Because it would be a nice thing for you to do.' Your chance of getting what you want is not great. Sound familiar? Working from home may be a new way of working, but it's the same process that each of us accept that we have to go through in order to get a job. If you reframe this *new* thing in to a *familiar* thing, then suddenly it's not such a big deal and it feels achievable.

So, let's get started. When you are looking to arrange a working from home role with your employer I would say that it is important to approach this as if you are proposing outsourcing the current service provider (old you) to a better service provider (new you): The key word being *better*. Even if you don't present it in these literal terms, it's still a good idea to approach it in this way in order that you can objectify the situation and look to identify what the needs are, so you can establish how you can fulfil those needs. I would recommend approaching it as if you are a separate company and your boss is your client. You are looking to win the business from that client. Why would that client go with you? What are you offering that is better than what they currently have? What is your USP (unique selling point?) However, be mindful not to condemn their current service provision too much; because remember that's you.

Take action

Without doubt the most important ingredient in bringing this change about is to take action. You can hypothesise and speculate the outcome of this as much as you like but unless you take action then nothing will ever happen, and you will never know what might have been. We pretty much all know this to be true, but it doesn't make it any easier or any less nerve-wracking for when the time finally comes for you to take the required action.

Many of us will buy a book or watch a TV show and be really inspired and motivated by it. 'Ok, that's it. I'm going to change my life', we say. What happens next? The passion and emotional charge begins to fade and those little voices of doubt start whispering. Before long those whispers have turned in to fully articulated reasons why you could never do it. This is a common scenario for many of us and the outcome is all too often that we give in to those doubts straight away and don't follow through with the ideas that have inspired us.

I would encourage you to not give in to those early doubts that you'll be hearing. However, I would also discourage you from ignoring them totally. Instead, I would suggest you involve them in the process. When you have done your due diligence and established that it is indeed something that is right for you, and balanced your motivations against your doubts; then you can really begin in earnest to make it happen. Taking the action required on this solid foundation of objectivity will give you a much stronger chance of success than a flimsy emotional reaction to a short-lived fantasy.

Negotiating a working from home role with my boss
I had never even heard about working from home back when I first spoke to my boss about my relocating. It was simply that we had the opportunity to come to Australia and I had to tell my boss that I would be leaving. It was he that originally suggested that we consider the idea of my staying with the company and work remotely. However once he'd suggested the idea, I was very keen to make this happen and I quickly set about doing all I could to make it a reality. The more I considered it, the more I thought it was a great idea. I

really enjoyed my job, and one of the less appealing consequences of our moving was that I would have to leave my job and find another one. I also really liked the industry that I was working in but, realistically, jobs in that sector are generally located in major cities. Our primary motivation for moving was lifestyle and I didn't much like the idea of swapping one busy commuter train for another one in a different part of the world. This idea of working from home could really offer the perfect solution for us.

Once he'd put the idea out there it was then up to me to really sell it in to him and to the company. I was essentially applying for a new role with the company, but one where there was no job description and no precedents that I could use as comparables. I needed to both define the role and convince my boss that I was the man for the job.

I set about putting a pitch together, using the same methods we would use when we pitched to other companies for their business; by identifying the opportunity (what the needs were) and demonstrating why I was the right man for them (how I could fulfil those needs). This process involved me objectively looking at myself as an employee and what I brought to the table. What was unique about me and why should they take a punt on me, rather than take the easy option and get a new 'me'? What were my USPs?

I am not being modest when I say that I am not a particularly gifted individual. I am simply being honest and would say that, in my professional experience, very few people are unusually gifted or irreplaceable. In terms of our skill sets, we're all pretty interchangeable as is evidenced when an employee leaves and is replaced by somebody else. A job description is written, outlining the skill set required, a replacement is hired and business resumes as usual.

The main thing that differentiates us as employees is our personality and our attitude, and how these are deployed in the workplace. Since I had joined the company I had set up a small team and managed that team pretty well. My boss had confidence in me as a manager. He knew that I understood the deliverables required and that I would make sure my team delivered the work on time and to the quality required. Very good, however the remote role that we were looking at did not involve managing a team and did not require me to be a good people person. I would be working alone and not in charge of a team of people. Regardless, I set about explaining the importance of this experience, in that I understood work-streams and could be depended upon to deliver the work on time and to the expected standards and, although it was only me, I was still managing a team - just a team of one.

Probably the main reasons that my boss decided to keep me on, in the end, was the knowledge that I had. I had set up work systems and had intimate knowledge of our clients and their needs. This would not be impossible to replace, as the new employee would simply learn it all themselves, but it would take time and it would advantageous for them to keep me and retain that knowledge base.

Another reason that he kept me on was that I had

experience in client pitches and so, although it wasn't my core specialism, I could also look to develop a client base in the region.

The final reason was that I could work for less money. The cost of living was lower in Australia and this, together with my duties being less, meant that they could retain my services at a much cheaper rate.

As a summary:
- I had management skills that would be useful in managing my 'team of one'
- I had intimate knowledge of internal systems and client needs that would be good to retain
- I could develop our business in the region, in an additional capacity
- I could work for substantially less money

It took some research and discussion and after a few weeks an agreement was reached that myself and my deputy would essentially swap jobs, with him becoming my boss and assuming the team management responsibilities. He was somebody that I had worked with for many years, both at this company and at my previous one. We knew each other extremely well and I thought this to be the perfect solution. My contract was for an initial six months and would be reviewed after that. If it didn't work out then this time period would have at least served as a transition and I could help with a successful handover. I was to be paid my new salary as gross in UK currency and it would be down to me to transfer that in to Australian currency each month, and to pay my income tax in Australia. We had a contract drawn up that named me as 'General Manager,

Australia' and I was very happy with this package that we had put together.

Define your performance metrics

A very important thing that I would recommend you take some time to do at this stage is to define your performance metrics. One of the things that working from home radically challenges is how our efficiency is managed and recorded. With a remote worker not being there in the office, it is not easy for their manager to see that they are actually working. Our conventional way of measuring an employee's efficiency is to see how many hours they are sitting at their desk although, as we know, this is not an accurate indicator of how much work is actually getting done.

It's not always easy for businesses to measure *output* and so, instead, *input* is often focused on as the performance metric. For example, if somebody does the same amount of work in four days as it takes another to do in six days, then it will be the latter that is best received as he worked all week, and even put in a day at the weekend. This is a way of thinking that is difficult to shift in all of us.

It's not surprising that input is often judged more than output as, without accurate metrics for measurement, much of this judgment happens on a subconscious level. Let's look at a scenario of three workers who all produce identical output, but have different levels of input: if I am a manager and I see employee one in the office every day, then I will think of them as 'dependable'. If I see employee two there in the office every day and some evenings as well, then I think of them as 'committed'. If I do not see employee three there (as they are a remote worker) then subconsciously I may not feel that they are as committed or dependable as the rest of my team, although their productivity is exactly the same. While it is useful to recognise that this situation may exist, it is important to understand that, as it happens on a subconscious level, it is not intentional and so try not to take it personally.

As children, we have a simplistic view that there are employees and *the boss*. The reality is, in most companies, everybody has a boss and you have to go a long way up the chain of command before you get to the 'big boss,' and even he or she potentially has bosses in the form of share-holders. We are all accountable to somebody else and, as a remote worker, your boss will need to have a good handle on your efficiency levels in order to report to their boss (who in turn reports to theirs and so it goes on). Having been a manager myself I definitely found it was much easier for me to understand what my manager would want to see from me in terms of efficiency and productivity. I understood that he wasn't asking because he was judging me or wanted to give me a hard time but simply because my accountability to him was directly related to his accountability to his boss, and so on.

By taking some time to define the ways which your performance will be judged, you'll be giving yourself and your boss a measurable gauge with which to determine your output levels. This should enable you to have a better understanding of what is expected of you and some objective accountability. It'll also provide you with some targets to beat, with your work-time now being more focused and productive.

CHAPTER SUMMARY

Assuming the role of a company to a client is a good way to approach arranging a working from home role with your employer, as it will help you to objectify the situation and identify the needs required.

What do you currently provide that your boss would not want to lose? What is unique to you?

Define your performance metrics with your boss.

Take action. Nothing will happen without you taking the action required to bring it about.

9. MAKING THE MOVE

'The secret of getting ahead is getting started'
Agatha Christie

So at last, the time had finally come for us to make our big move. Angela and I had decided that the way to make the strongest start was for her and the kids to go out first and get everything set up. In that time I would continue working in the office and make sure that the transition was as seamless as possible. When she had everything set up then I would follow them out and begin working as soon as possible. This made a lot of sense from a practical perspective, but it did mean that she was flying to the other side of the world with a baby and two small children all by herself. Then when she arrived, she would have to buy a car, rent a house, get the kids in to school, set up phones, taxes and the list goes on. We decided that three weeks would be a good time period to work to and so, she had a three week deadline to achieve all of this.

At the time, Florence was ten, Alice was six and Michael was eighteen months old. Florence really 'stepped up to the plate' during this time and was an invaluable second in command. She was a huge asset to Angela and we were very proud of the way she took on all of these new challenges with such enthusiasm and maturity. This was the beginning of our new chapter and we were all working together.

My arrival

When it came time for me to fly out it was very strange for me to be making the journey on my own. My family and I were moving to the other side of the world. We had been planning it for a long time, but now the time had finally arrived and it seemed odd that it was just me on that plane. It had been a very good move for me to stay back and make sure that the transition with work was as seamless as we could make it. It had also been good that Angela and the kids came out first and set everything up from that end. The move was being facilitated by my work and so work had to be the priority - in establishing a solid set of foundations with my work, we were giving ourselves the best possible chance for success in all other areas. Although we had agreed this course of action together, and I knew it was the right thing to do, I couldn't help feeling a bit lazy and that she had the bulk of the work to do all by herself and here I was sitting on my own enjoying interruption free movies on the plane.

Since they had left I had spoken to Angela regularly and knew that everything was going well and I also knew her well enough to know that she would revel in the challenges that she was presented with. Sure enough, by the time I arrived with my laptop in hand we had a car, a home, the kids were in school and my laptop was ready to connect to the UK server and start work straight away - I am married to Wonder woman!

Angela met me at the airport with baby Michael and whisked me straight off to the city to sign endless bits of paper, before picking up the two girls from school. I had really missed everybody and seeing our beautiful girls in their new school uniforms come out of the classrooms with huge beaming smiles was such a welcome sight. They told me all about what had happened and just couldn't get the words out quick enough. When you go to a different place on holiday, everything about it appears different; it smells different, looks different and feels different. That's what it was like for me when I first arrived. It felt like I was on an amazing holiday and everything was new and exciting - except that my family were my travel guides. They were living there and already seemed so happy and settled in their new environment; all within just three weeks.

I had a couple of days to get settled and get over my jet-lag before starting work. I spent this time being shown around my new life by my family. It was the middle of summer, the sun was shining and it was such a strange but exciting time, especially as I had just come from a freezing mid-winter in the UK. My deadline for arriving was Florence's birthday. She is a Valentine's Day baby and I arrived the day before and made sure that I was fully recharged by then. The plan was that we would celebrate her birthday going to an outdoor Valentines concert with our new friends that evening. This was my first introduction to such events and I loved it. It was a hot night and we sat under the stars on our picnic blanket and enjoyed a great evening of entertainment. I will never forget this event and how it served as an introduction to this wonderful new lifestyle.

Our first overseas office

All of our belongings had to be shipped over which took two months, so during that time we had no furniture at all in our house. We slept on the floors and we bought a fold-up plastic picnic table for me to work on. This served as our family meal table and my office, until our furniture arrived. The company I work for now has International offices all over the world but, back then, our little red fold-up picnic table was our first overseas office. After breakfast each day, the spilt milk would be wiped away and the table would be moved upstairs to the room that I worked in. After work each day, the laptop would duly be put away and the table would then be carried down to the kitchen to become the dinner table. We knew the furniture was on its way so, managing like this for a short time, was never a problem. We would sometimes go to the port where the container ships arrived and the kids would see the hundreds of containers being craned on to the dock and ask which one was ours.

If the desk itself wasn't a great office then the view I had certainly made up for it. Angela had surpassed herself and managed to rent us a two storey house with amazing views out on to the Indian Ocean. Each morning I would wave goodbye to Angela and the kids from the balcony, as they walked to school. When I went back inside to start work I would marvel at the beautiful view of the Indian Ocean that was the backdrop of my working day.

It's a big deal!

Angela and I are both positive people and we are firm in the belief that whatever attitudes you project yourself, are the exact same attitudes that your kids will adopt for themselves. We knew that moving to the other side of the world was something that the kids could have potentially been quite unnerved by and so we always played down its significance. 'It's not a big deal' we would say. A surprizing thing that occurred early on was that, we'd done such a good job telling the kids that it wasn't a big deal that we'd come to believe it ourselves. Now we were on the other side of the world and away from our safe and comfortable world, we adults suddenly felt overwhelmed by what we had done and thought: 'Aargh, it's a big deal!' Everybody asked how the kids were settling in and, had the same assumptions that we had; that the kids would be the ones that needed time and encouragement settling in to their new environment. What we discovered was the opposite. The kids were fine because they had everything structured for them. They had left their school structure in the UK and simply moved to a different structure somewhere else. They had no concept of the fact that it was on the other side of the planet. They weren't exposed to all of the endless grown up stuff required and were just busy getting on with the job of being a kid. The children were fine but we adults were, privately, pretty freaked out for a while.

Business as usual

Work began well for me. There were one or two teething problems that my London colleague and I worked through together. We had worked together for so many years that we knew each other well and were a great team. One early bonus that we discovered, that we hadn't fully considered before was the time difference. With my working Australian hours, we were now able to provide a twenty four hour service. People were coming in to the London office the next morning to find the work they'd requested all done. We would joke that it was like the children's fairy-tale; 'The Elves and the Shoemaker', where each morning the shoemaker would awake to discover that during the night magic elves had made perfect pairs of shoes for him to sell in his shop that day.

Our daughters' school lives were going well. It was all very different for them and it was exciting for us to listen to them tell of their new experiences. Every morning they raised the national flag, they sung the national anthem in assembly and sang hymns in chapel; this was all very different to their previous school life in the UK. They had made friends and were doing very well with their studies, particularly Alice the younger of the two. Our eldest daughter Florence has always been academically very strong whereas it has never come so easy for Alice, who had to have extra lessons at times to try and keep up in the UK. In her new school she was blossoming. It was now February and the start of a new Australian academic year and, because the school calendar ends in July in the UK (and begins again in September), she was a full term ahead of the work they were learning. The work that she was being taught was work she knew already and so, for the first time, she was at the top of the class. This early lift in confidence and perception really turned things around for her and she has never looked back; doing well ever since.

Children's school calendars are an important thing to consider when looking at potential dates to make a move. Having the opportunity to get our kids 'ahead of the curve' academically worked out very well for us.

CHAPTER SUMMARY

This is when it all becomes real. You are strapped in to that rollercoaster and there is no turning back now.

Consider the time of year you will be starting out in. Seeing your new environment in the best possible light will give you a stronger motivation to make the move a success. Also, look for opportunities to get 'ahead of the curve' such as school calendars.

Working from home puts a greater dependency on the reliability and efficiency of the technology that we rely on to make it work. It's important to do adequate due diligence in this area.

DANIEL BOND

10. NEW EXPERIENCES

'The dog that trots about finds a bone'
Golda Meir

In the early days, there were so many things that were new and exciting for us. Different accents, climate, money, wildlife, environment: Different everything. Like all things, you quickly learn to take them in to your stride and before you know it the unknown is suddenly the known. We have so many stories that we have recounted over the years but here some experiences of our stumbling upon some of these different things when they were all new and exciting.

These are just a taste of some of the new things that we've enjoyed together and are exactly the sort of experiences that we imagined all those years ago when we were contemplating relocating. What sort of memories do you want to look back on? Where in the world would these take place? What sort of activities would you be doing and who would you be doing them with? Working back from 'future memories' is a good way to begin thinking about how you can make them happen.

New wildlife

One thing I still love about the environment that I'm lucky enough to live and work in is the wildlife. I love it that while I'm working in my home office, I can hear all of the different variety of parrots in the trees in our garden. I always love seeing pelicans and am still constantly amazed when they actually get off the ground. They are so big (they're like a dog with wings) and I wonder how they can ever fly. I love hearing the kookaburra (sounding like a jungle monkey) and I love the morning chorus of birds when we are in the bush. I love seeing kangaroos on the golf course (not caring if somebody is under par or over par) and I love seeing the dolphins and rays in the ocean.

In this part of Australia, koala bears were hunted to extinction many years ago so they are no longer native here, but there is a colony relocated in a national park near where we live. As koalas are not the most active of creatures during daytime, in the early days, we created a game where we would get points for seeing them do certain things. They are generally asleep in the trees and are not always easy to spot, so there is a basic ten points awarded for each one spotted. Whoever spots one awake is awarded twenty points and, if they are walking to another tree or climbing, then that's the big fifty points.

One day, when we hadn't lived here long, we saw something that was off the points scale. We saw a koala bear fight. We've still never found anybody else that's seen such a thing but it's definitely one of the funniest sights I've ever witnessed in the natural world. Two koala bears were very close to each other on the same tree and one of them suddenly fell on top of the other one, which caused this bear to awaken and produce the strangest angry sound. The aggrieved bear then took a swipe at the other one and then promptly fell asleep. What followed was like a koala Rocky movie with both bears fighting angrily but then falling asleep in between punches. One would take a swipe at the other and be so exhausted by the activity that they'd promptly fall asleep again, only to be woken by receiving a blow and remembering that they were angry and involved in a fight. It was great fun to watch and was a bit like watching two feisty old pensioners going toe to toe and falling asleep between punches. It lasted for about ten minutes until eventually, exhausted by the bout, neither bear came back from their sleep. This was definitely one to remember and was probably worth a few thousand points.

Another early experience we had with Australian wildlife was when we were driving back from a long trip and, after about five hours on the same long straight road, we saw a road house and decided to pull over for a break. As the roadhouse approached, it seemed to be moving and I assumed it was a heat haze but, as we got closer, we saw that it was a moving pattern of green and yellow. There were hundreds of thousands of green and yellow budgerigars covering the building and everything around it. We stopped and got out and waded through the sea of birds to the road house where the owners told us that the budgies had come in from the dessert in search of water, as it was so dry. It was over fifty degrees at the time and the sheer weight of the birds had broken a large tree branch, which had collapsed on to the generator. We stayed for a while and then upon leaving they asked the kids, jokingly, if they wanted a budgie. The kids all wanted one but as we were still two days drive from home we couldn't, as the birds would be dead by the time we got home.

Driving away, we had to have one person standing by each wheel, trying to usher the budgies out from under the car, as I reversed slowly out on to the road. Even doing this as carefully as possible we still had squashed budgies all over our car tyres as we drove away. Sitting in the back seat, we had a chorus of 'I want a budgie, I want a budgie..'. While we were driving I noticed that there was a 'willy willy' (a small red sand tornado you get in the bush) over to our right that was getting closer and closer. I slowed down to avoid and it slowed down. I sped up and it sped up. This went for a while until it became obvious that our paths would inevitably cross. Still the chorus of 'I want a budgie' continued until suddenly the whole car was engulfed in dark red earth and we couldn't see a thing. The willy willy had hit us and it was like being shaken around in a sand car wash at 110kph. The lights went out for what seemed like ages (though it was just probably a matter of seconds) and I did my best to carry on driving straight on. Suddenly it was gone and we were back in bright daylight. There was silence throughout the car as everybody wondered what on earth had just happened. Nobody said anything for a long time and we thought the kids might be too terrified to speak, after what they had just been through. Then suddenly, with no word about what had just happened, they began chorusing; 'I want a budgie, I want a budgie...'

They never did get their budgie but we always smile

whenever we see one in a pet shop.

New accents

One of the great things about travel is the exposure to different types of people and their different ways of talking. When we had only been living here a short time we were still becoming accustomed to hearing different accents. When our son was little, we were walking along in a ferry terminal on one occasion and there was a New Zealand family alongside us. The Dad was looking to get his family booked in for the ferry and was saying aloud 'Where's the check-in?' My son heard him and started looking around on the floor. The more the man repeated, 'Where's the check-in?' the harder our little Michael looked around. After a few minutes he looked up at me and said, confused; 'What chicken?'

Park life

We had many great experiences with the 'big' differences, but having three young kids, much of our life was taken up doing the 'little' things and we spent a lot of our early days in children's play parks. The parks here all have sand on the ground and shade sails above, to take the brightness out of the sun rays. They are well maintained and the kids run around bare-foot in their shorts and sun-hats. These parks were a real pleasure to spend time in and still are, although we do not have to clock-up so many hours in them these days.

The atmosphere in the parks in England, mainly due to the weather, was very different. When the weather was good, these places would be so crowded that the kids would often have to wait their turn to go on things. When the weather wasn't so good, the apparatus would often be so wet that the kid's clothes would get soaked or it'd sometimes be so cold that it wasn't much fun to be there for long.

Our youngest daughter Alice has always been a real chatterbox and we would spend hours pushing her on the swings while she chatted away about one thing or another, while we pushed her. On one occasion in England, I had been pushing her on a swing for forty five minutes while she chatted away happily. It was a freezing cold afternoon, we were the only people in the park and, as it was getting dark, I decided it was time to go home. I stopped the swing for her to get off but she couldn't move her hands. They were so cold that they were locked in position griping the swing. It was literally so cold that I was genuinely worried that her skin had frozen to the metal of the swings. For forty five minutes she had been happily chatting away about her favourite stuff and nonsense and now she'd stopped, she realised that she was cold. As I began to slowly unpeel her fingers and hands from the metal she cried out from the cold. Finally we got her hands free and hurried home to warm up.

We have recollected this memory a few times when we have happily been enjoying some family time at the park, and it all seems like a distant memory now.

Big blue sky
One of the first things that struck us when we were first here is how 'big' the sky was. I know it sounds crazy, as I'm sure the sky is the same size everywhere but it just felt bigger. Coming from the UK where everything is packed together in the towns and cities and, even in the

country, there are always forests or hillsides to break up the horizon. Add to this the seemingly constant low cloud base that hangs over the UK most of the time, and you sometimes feel that you never really see the sky or the horizon. Sometimes when you're landing in an aeroplane in the UK, you start the descent and are plunged in to thick cloud. These thick layers of cloud last for a long time and just when you get out of the cloud and expect to look down and see the ground far below, you're landing. The cloud is almost to the ground.

For much of the year here, the sky is very clear. So much so that, statistically, it has one of best records for clear skies and so quite a few Asian airlines have training schools based here. Also, apart from the city, the buildings are quite low and the terrain is very flat. These things combined really give you a sense of the sky being 'bigger' and, nowhere more so, than out in the bush.

When our dog Biscuit was a very small puppy we were away camping at a remote homestead in the bush. For miles around all you could see was low level bush-land scrub. No trees, no real hills of any note and a huge blue sky up top. When we were packing up to go home, our little puppy went under the car, as this was the only shade available now that the tent had been taken down. We finally got everything packed in to the car but, as we hadn't had him very long, we completely forgot about our puppy.

We drove off out of the homestead, up the bitumen track and back to the road. We were about twenty minutes in to the long journey home when we suddenly realised that we had left our dog behind. The kids were distraught. We raced back to the homestead as quickly as possible, terrified about the possibilities of what we may find. It was a hot day with no shade and he could have wandered off anywhere to find shade. There were snakes out there. There were eagles, and he was a decent sized snack. Any number of possibilities ran through our minds as we drove back, racked with guilt about what bad dog owners we were.

When we got back we were faced with this huge expanse of land, topped with this huge expanse of sky and one tiny little puppy sitting in exactly the same spot as we had left him. We were so relieved and expecting a huge and grateful welcome, like something from a Lassie movie, he just looked at us as if to say 'oh, there you are', and we picked him up and put him in the car. Big sky; big land; huge relief.

Christening a new life
One great experience that we had in those early days in Australia, was actually in England. We came back for our first visit after we had been living there for just over six months. Life was great and we were filled with optimism about our new chapter down under, but were looking forward to coming back and seeing friends and family and telling them all about our adventures so far. As part of this trip we had also planned to have our son christened while we were there. It took some planning, as we were out of the parish area of all English churches and we had to plan it and invite all of our friends and family.

The day came and it was a beautiful ceremony in a beautiful English church, followed by a great reception in a nearby pub. One of the wonderful things that you appreciate about the UK, when you live overseas is its architecture, and particularly the countless ancient churches that fill the landscape with their spires. We appreciated the ceremony even more for its historical venue and its formal and traditional setting. All of our friends and family were gathered together and it was great to see everybody. We were loving living under the hot sun on the other side of the world but really appreciated a cloudy day in an old English church, surrounded by family and friends even more for the contrast that it brought to these exciting times.

CHAPTER SUMMARY

What sort of memories do you want to make?

What do these memories consist of? Deconstructing 'future memories' is a good way to begin constructing a pathway towards them.

Our memories are not only from exploring our new environment, but also from gaining a positive appreciation of our previous one.

11. EXPERIENCING PROBLEMS

'If you can meet with Triumph and Disaster
And treat those two impostors just the same'
Extract from 'If' by Rudyard Kipling

At some point after you have started working from home you will inevitably experience problems. I am not being pessimistic, it is simply that problems come along at all times in our lives and we have to deal with them. The same will happen when you are working remotely, only the nature of your new remote setting may make these problems feel magnified. In the past you may have had a support network in the office to help you deal with work problems. You've probably had a support network (in the form of family and friends) to help you out with problems outside of work. These networks are now gone and experiencing problems may feel slightly different as a result of this.

Our introduction to this new chapter in our lives could not have gone better. We were very happy with our new surroundings and were really enjoying the moment, but we were about to hit our first major problem that would change things dramatically.

Angela and I had both worked hard in ensuring that we had enough money to really maximise our new lifestyle in Australia. We wanted to release ourselves from enough financial burdens in order that that we could really enjoy our new life and the extra time that we would have to spend with our family. She had been running a successful business for over twenty years and I had been fortunate enough to have enjoyed a career that paid me well. We had never been extravagant with money and had never lived in a huge money-pit of a house. Instead we always had a comfortable house, with a comfortable financial cushion that allowed us to have great holidays and regular weekends away. 'Little house, big life' we always said. This modest lifestyle meant that, together with the sale of our property, we had reached the target amount of what we were aiming for. We had enough money to potentially allow us to buy a nice home, with a swimming pool, without having to take out a mortgage.

Although I was really happy with my work, as I have said previously, at first it was viewed by the company as a 'work-in-progress' and we really didn't know how long I would be able to continue to work remotely. My longer term plan was actually to get my Commercial Pilot's License and fly tourist/bush flights and, later, some instructing. I had been flying as a hobby for many years and always loved the idea of doing it for a job but, unless you are working for an airline, then it really is more of a vocation than a career - it doesn't pay well and the work is sporadic. Due to her commitments to her business, Angela had also felt that she had missed out on too much of the girls' childhood. As she had a business partner, she was able to share the responsibility and so neither of them had to work full-time hours. She was always grateful to have had a good balance between work and motherhood but, with our youngest Michael; she was determined that she wanted to be a full-time Mum and to fully appreciate the joys of motherhood, as it would be her last time. She was happy to work again once our youngest had started school, but she definitely wasn't interested in starting another business and living through the stresses and strains of being a business owner again. We had factored these desires in to our plan and, part of the goal of building up our wealth level was so that we would be able to fulfil these goals.

It is at this part of the story that our life changed forever. About a year before we left, we sold our property and rented a house. Angela had just given birth to Michael and we were not ready to commit to the move just yet, and so we spent the next twelve months living quite happily and had banked the funds from our house sale. Life was good and we were very happy with our lot, plus we had the opportunity of our relocation to look forward to in the future.

As we were not going anywhere for a while, we decided to invest our money with my Father-in-law. He is a charming and likeable man with great stories, great charisma but a history of broken marriages and broken promises. We always enjoyed a good relationship with him, because we accepted the way he was, flaws and all, and so never placed ourselves in a vulnerable position with him. He lived in South Africa where the rules of conduct in business are often 'flexible' and he and his friendship group did very well for themselves.

When we transferred our money to him on a Friday we instantly realised that we had made a mistake, but we would now have to wait until Monday to organise the return of these funds. We had forgotten why our relationship was successful and we had, for the first time, placed ourselves in a vulnerable position. The day after we had transferred the funds (Saturday), he suffered a stroke and had instructed the office in South Africa to tell us that our money had already been invested and that it would be locked up for three months. We reluctantly accepted that we would have to wait three months, especially as he would be spending some time recovering in hospital.

Time went by and we were persistently asking for our money to be returned to us but, what we didn't realise is that, while he had access to our money he had decided to use it to 'prop up' a property deal in Cape Town. He hadn't invested it for us as he had said, but had used it for something that he believed to be 'a sure thing'. He figured that he would use our money as capital, make a quick buck and put the capital back without us even knowing. When it came to light what he had done we were furious, but we had zero control and there really was nothing we could do. The deal was with one of his oldest friends and he vouched for his credibility – indeed, he also had a lot of his own money tied up in it. We had it agreed that we would have it all returned plus interest, before we left for Australia.

I'm sure you can guess where this is going; probably at the outset most people would have guessed, but we naively believed that our money would be returned to us, with interest. The money didn't come back before we left for Australia but we were assured that it was 'on its way'. Angela could not believe that her Father would not return our money, it was inconceivable.

Our arrival in Australia coincided with a 'once in a generation' economic boom. China was a rapidly growing economy that wanted Australia's natural resources as quickly as they could dig it up. Prices were high, business was booming, the population was expanding and property prices were going through the roof. Every day that we were without our money saw further increases in property prices. Meanwhile, we were still being told that it was 'on its way' and had no choice other than to wait and hope.

We were viewing properties to purchase, within our price range and one day we saw one that we wanted to buy, but were told that we would have to match an existing offer there and then. Properties were selling themselves and real estate agents were enjoying heady days. We phoned my Father-in-law and told him that we could secure the property but would have to take out a 'bridging loan' (a very high interest temporary loan) until our money arrived - when would it be here? At this point he finally told us for the first time that he wouldn't be able to repay us anytime soon, and that it was probably best if we didn't take on a bridging loan.

We had made our first mistake in forgetting why we had always enjoyed a healthy relationship with him. Our second mistake was in assuming that, when family was involved, he would act differently to his instincts. He made the mistake of assuming that his 'friend' would act differently to his instincts.

In to Africa

My Father-in-Law gave us the phone number of his 'friend' who endlessly told us that he was sorry that we were caught up in a difficult situation and the money was 'tied up' but that he would do what he could for us (we later discovered that he had actually transferred some of our money back to us via my Father-in-law who had taken it for himself, while we were already in Australia and desperate for our money). He had had a bitter fall out with my Father-in-law, which ended up in legal dealings and we were still no further forward. While all of this was going on, property prices had gone up so much that, even if we got our money back tomorrow, then we could never afford the type of house that we had planned. House prices had risen over 25% in the time that we had been without our money.

We felt desperate and had to do something and so Angela, together with our baby, went out to South Africa to try and resolve the situation. I stayed back with the girls and carried on with business as usual. This trip procured little, apart from some memorable experiences of the seedier aspects of her Father's life in South Africa. She and her Father sat in endless meetings with his lawyer. She witnessed some of her Father's dealings with a 'colourful' ex-policeman, who was 'flexible' in his distribution of justice. His 'justice' was basically dispensed on behalf of the highest bidder and, they later discovered that as well as talking to my Father-in-law, he was also having the same conversations with his former 'friend' (now enemy) who was also courting him for his services. She also witnessed how her Father's financial situation was a total mess that matched that of our own. He also had all of his money 'invested', plus he had never fully recovered from his stroke and his eye-sight and memory faculties were severely impaired. On one occasion he had to 'de-stress' and so his driver took him to his latest favourite prostitute, while Angela and baby Michael waited in the car outside with his driver.

After a short time it became clear that it was a lost cause and there was nothing else that she could do. She had explored every avenue and so returned home empty handed. We finally had to resign ourselves to the fact that we would never see our money again. With this knowledge we at least felt some closure and knew that we would need to get on with our lives without it.

Next...
When things are going badly all of us are sensitive to looking out for the next bad thing. We had been enjoying a great run of things going our way and had probably taken them for granted. There had undoubtedly been a great many blessings come our way over recent times but we had just taken them on board without too much notice. Now that we were experiencing a run of loses (as everybody does, from time to time) we were terrified of the next bit of bad news to land at our doorstep. We had lost our life savings (and it was no small amount of money) but, this combined with being left out of a 'once in a generation' property boom, meant that our financial misfortune had being accelerated and we were feeling out of control. Our net worth was pretty much at zero and we thought we couldn't go any lower. We were wrong.

Angela's hairdressing salon had been a great business

for over twenty years. She had run it together with her business partner who is also one of her best friends. Sadly, Angela lost her mother many years ago and her business partner became more like family. Neither of them wanted the salon to be anything other than what it was; a modest reliable, local and friendly salon that was as much a meeting place for old friends as anything else. They had lots of regulars who they knew well and were familiar with their lives and the lives of their children and grandchildren. Their clients loved the modest, comfortable and friendly atmosphere and they also appreciated the good value that they would get. Angela and her partner never had any aspirations to turn it in to a high priced, trendy salon with loud music and cappuccinos. They knew their market and knew what their needs were. It was a good steady business that made good, if not amazing, profits.

At the same time that our financial ship was sinking, Angela was told by her business partner that the free-holders had changed at the shop. They had both known the couple who had owned the property for many years and they always gave them a good deal, as they knew that it was a good little business that was valued by the community. They had told them that, after all these years, they were selling the property but would put in a good word with the new free-holders. Unfortunately, the new owners were not interested in the value to the community and informed us that the rent would be doubling. There is no way that the business could survive with this added to the cash-flow sheet. Not only that but they also informed us that, they had taken legal advice and found that they were within their rights to backdate this rent. They would therefore be backdating the rent and we now potentially owed them a huge amount of money.

None of us had the money and, clearly, we were not in a position where we could take out a loan to pay them. We no longer had any assets and were living on the other side of the world. The business would have to close and we would have to try and find the money to pay redundancy bills for several members of staff, plus this apparent debt that we now owed. Angela's partner was left with the task of; finding the legal position with lawyers, the financial position with their accountant, having the business valued and trying to negotiate with the new free-holders. The highest of highs that we had felt so recently, with the start of this exciting new chapter, were now replaced by the lowest of lows.

CHAPTER SUMMARY

Try and avoid being swept up too much in the optimism of your new life change and become careless.

Inevitable problems will occur from time to time just as they do at other times in life, but they may feel magnified with your remote situation.

At times of difficulty you may feel especially isolated with distance between you and your support network.

Your new remote setting can make you feel overwhelmed by your problems and it is often easy to forget all of the good fortune that you may have had.

12. DEALING WITH PROBLEMS

**'There are costs and risks to a program of action,
but they are far less than the long range risks and
costs of comfortable inaction'**
John F Kennedy

When you are working from home you will experience inevitable problems that you will need to deal with yourself. With your support network gone, there is no hiding place and you will need to resolve the problem yourself. To use a literal metaphor of remoteness; in the past your car may have broken down and so you either phoned your auto-recovery service or perhaps somebody from your support network (such as your Dad or a good friend who can fix cars) came to help you out and get you home again. Your new remote situation is comparable to having your car break-down on a lonely isolated stretch of road that is out of range for auto-recovery services and for anybody to come and help you. You *need* to fix the car yourself. This may be daunting for you but it is all part of taking responsibility for your decision to take that route. These inevitable problems are tests and a necessary part of your journey in to the unknown.

With the situation that we had found ourselves in it felt like our *dream* was over, but the reality was that our *real life* was just beginning. Fantasy had to give way to reality and, no matter how hard we wished, we would wake up in the morning and the situation would still be the same. The dream life that we had focused so hard on was not on the menu anymore and it was a salvage operation. Angela dealt with this much better than I did. She is the practical one and knew that, like it or not, we needed to get on to the property ladder at whatever level we could afford in order to house our family. We were finding it hard to pay the rent now and had to trim our life to our new means. Thankfully we had put some money aside to help us get established and this money was basically enough to either get us and our furniture back to the UK or to put a small deposit down on a property. We had the choice of going back broke and, literally, starting over again or sticking it out here and seeing what the future had in store for us. We decided to stay and gaining dual Citizenship was our goal now, for all of our futures. Going back beaten was not an option. Our goal was to survive and prosper and the first part of surviving meant having somewhere to live and work.

A new reality
This new reality was not easy to accept but it was crunch time and decisions had to be made. There was a long period of time where I was filled with so much furious anger and self-pity. But we had to accept this new reality, deal with it and move forward. We did ultimately adapt, survive and move on and, it may sound crazy but, in many ways losing our life savings was the best thing that ever happened to us.

Angela found us a property that we could afford, with a huge mortgage. It was essentially a large dark brick shed in which a reclusive elderly lady had recently passed away in. Angela explained that we could renovate it and then move on to something bigger. At this time I was so busy feeling sorry for myself that I simply agreed and we moved in. Our youngest two kids thought it all a great adventure but Florence, who had left her great friends, great life and great home in England, sobbed her heart out. 'Not the black house!' she cried in a puddle of tears.

On our first night in the house, Angela and I were awoken by the sounds of screaming. Outside in the street, we discovered that one of our immediate neighbours was having a fight with his girlfriend. This kept us awake for much of the night thinking what on earth had we done, and this certainly didn't help improve our first impression of our new home. For a long time I was filled with rage with the injustice of what had happened to us. My pride had been hurt so much and I felt responsible and so wretched that I had let everybody down. I couldn't ignore it and the more I wallowed in that anger the more it consumed me. I awoke each morning to see our kids covered in sweat and insect bites from the holes in the roof and my heart would break.

I knew I had to be bigger. I had to remember all that we had learned from relocating in the first place; that the kids will be mirrors of our own feelings and behaviour. I had to dig deep and muster the feeling of hope and opportunity that this house and this life represented. If I continued down the track of self-pity and anger then this would simply be collectively adopted by the whole family and that behaviour that would consume us all. I had a responsibility to these little people in my life that went way beyond net worth. During this time Angela was the rock and I was letting her down too. I had to pull myself together and lead by example.

The work begins
'Necessity is the mother of invention' and so we set to work with the little resources we had at our disposal. The house didn't just need renovating in order for us to make money. It needed renovating to make it habitable for a family of five - that was the first task and we all set about it. There were only a few rooms and so we had to nominate which ones would be for the kids' bedrooms and, (as Angela and I were sleeping in the lounge) we had to repurpose the hallway to be a make-shift lounge room/office. The ceiling had exposed beams which meant there was no insulation and I had to constantly keep a fan on my laptop in order to keep it cool. The temperatures got up to nearly fifty degrees on occasion and one day I sat and watched a thick candle melt away over the course of my working day. As our youngest child was still a toddler, I often had to work with my pilot's head-set on, to block out the noises that all little people make throughout the day. One day while I was working, I felt something on my leg and looked down to see a red-back spider (which are potential deadly) crawling up towards my shorts. This was not something I had been used to dealing with in the London office.

The heat was always something to contend with and we spent most of our lives outside under shady areas. In order to gain side access to the property, I had to remove a wall which had a concrete soak-well in it (a soak-well is a huge concrete tube that funnels water down through the sand to the water table below). Removing a soak-well is a standard procedure that involves a machine for digging and a crane for removal. For budget purposes I had to do it all manually and, as it was so hot, I had to get up early in the morning and start digging before the day got too hot. Manually, this job required digging a huge hole and smashing the concrete soak-well with a sledgehammer (from within the hole) and bringing it up piece by piece. When the kids would get up for school and they'd ask Angela 'where's Daddy?' 'Here I am' I'd call from down my six foot hole and go and join them for breakfast before getting clean, logging on to the London server and starting my day's work.

Two months after moving in we had my sister-in-law and her two children come and visit us for our first Christmas in Australia. We had the TV in the hallway but the house wasn't big enough for the tree as well as the TV (we could only see half the screen) so the Christmas tree had to go outside. Before we had left the UK we had optimistically bought a large new Christmas tree for our large new house in Australia. Here we were having quite a different first Christmas than we had imagined and we had to laugh, when we remembered why we had bought that big tree. At that time my sister-in-law was unfortunately going through a very traumatic marriage break-up and so our tiny house was a hub of high emotions, five kids and a (not house trained) puppy.

We were having regular conversations with Angela's

business partner who was busily trying to resolve the situation back in the UK. It was a long process and we felt bad that she was burdened with having to deal with it all alone. She didn't mind and was, as ever, an absolute rock for us.

We had to try and earn extra money in order to fund the renovations and so we had to take on extra jobs. Because our youngest child was pre-school, Angela couldn't work full-time so she had to work in the evenings. I took on additional work that I juggled with my full-time job and meant me working some weekends. So, with Angela working every night, me working all day it seemed we barely saw each other. However, there were many hours that both of us would be working on the house together and, the plans that we had did need those extra funds.

At about this time Angela's Grandmother died. We were very sad, as we had been close; and even sadder because we couldn't be there to attend the funeral. The only good thing to come from this was that she had unexpectedly left us a small amount of money in her will, and so we swiftly put this money to good use in helping to fund our renovations. She would have been very proud of our efforts and happy that she was able to help us in a very meaningful way.

The outside of the house was scrub bush land and so we all mucked in and cleared it all. During this time we encountered a whole host of new and interesting wild life, some welcome and some not so welcome, such as poisonous snakes and spiders. (I should say here that, in the years that have past we have had very few experiences with the native snakes and spiders. They are definitely more afraid of us than we are of them, and they generally do whatever they can to keep out of our way. The renovation of this very old and run down property brought them all out from their homes, hence why we experienced so much of them at that time).We made tree swings, tree-houses, patio areas and pretty soon the garden was looking like a bush paradise. Every member of our family joined in to the big adventure of making a home out of this wild piece of unloved land. Michael, our youngest used to jump in to the hole that I was digging to bed the trampoline in (8ft x 5ft and 4ft deep) and, with his little bucket and spade, he used to flick sand around in an effort to help me with the digging (most of it just going all over me as I sweated in my labours). After lots of digging and using old doors for retaining the sand, the trampoline was finally in the hole. When we had friends over and were showing them the trampoline, Michael proudly declared to everybody: 'That's the hole that we dug isn't it Daddy.' We all laughed at the amount of actual *help* he'd been but really that statement made our hearts sing. It wasn't the work that went in to it, but rather the spirit of shared experience that had infused it. We were all mucking in and working together to move ourselves forward. It was fun. I was pushing the kids around in the wheel barrow, they were filthy most of the time, they carried rocks, painted walls and, when they weren't helping, they climbed trees and played in the sand. If they had sat inside on a computer game, waiting for the house to be done, then perhaps we would have different memories of that time, but they didn't. We had never been so proud of our family.

In little more than a year we had turned that little brick shed in to a beautiful cottage in its beachside location. We had knocked down walls and created new rooms, fitted a new kitchen, laid floorboards, rendered and painted the walls (inside and out), built a huge deck on the front, retiled the roof and made the garden in to a kid's adventure paradise. In the end, we didn't really want to leave - but there was no way that we could all squeeze in there for much longer.

We have such fond memories of that house, where we were always busy, either playing or working, until we all dropped at the end of the day. One day Michael was so exhausted from the heat of the day that he fell asleep, face down in his dinner bowl!

We took on the house that nobody wanted and turned it in to something that people did want - and we did it together. We sold that house and could afford to move to something much bigger and better, and we have lived there ever since. Our little family had turned our fortunes around together. We do not live in a palace, and we may never be able to afford that beautiful house with the pool that we dreamed of when we first arrived, but we have a great family home that we all worked together to get.

A healing time
In many ways renovating that old house was a metaphor for renovating our own lives. The changes taking place in the house represented the changes taking place in our hearts and minds. For the most part, our kids were oblivious to the change in our lives and in our circumstances, but they had every opportunity to

become dissatisfied and to complain about their lot. They were going to a private school and some of their friend's houses were beautiful mansions. Our eldest daughter Florence went to a school friend's house one day and got lost on the way back from going to the toilet – she had to call for somebody to come and find her. They could have easily have looked at their home and questioned why our house was different, but they didn't. They were just living day by day and enjoying whatever came their way. Angela and I could have simply blamed each other for our circumstances. I could have stayed wallowing in self-pity. We didn't – we all pulled together and there is no doubt that that experience made us all a much tighter family. Renovating that old house turned out to be the healing of us.

CHAPTER SUMMARY

There is no hiding place with a remote location. You need to take responsibility for the set of circumstances that have presented themselves. You need to own the problem.

Your relationships may be tested in difficult situations and good teamwork is paramount.

Difficult situations can be opportunities to learn about yourselves as individuals and as a family.

You need to remember why you are doing all of this. Remember the objectives you set and keep on course to achieving them.

Put these problems in an appropriate context. Your remoteness may make any problems feel overwhelming but they are simply tests in dealing with new situations outside of your comfort zone.

13. LEARNING FROM YOUR EXPERIENCES

'Very often a change of self is needed
more than a change of scene'
A. C. Benson

The situations you find yourself in may be difficult but eventually you will get through them. The real value in these experiences is what they teach you. To learn from them so that you can prepare yourself better and hopefully find ways of avoiding them in the future. The opportunity of working from home can teach you so much about yourself; not just how well you manage to work outside of the office environment. It is an opportunity to create new ways of living.

After we had dealt with our difficult financial situation we had to move on with our lives, but we could not have done so if we weren't willing to ask some uncomfortable questions of ourselves and to learn ways with which to deal with the unfavourable situation that we found ourselves in. This period of time taught us many things and these have not been forgotten but firmly adopted in the ways that we live to this day.

Owning the problem

We've all heard the self-help book adages before, but it's only when they resonate with your own life experience that they begin to make any sense to you. We knew the one about 'owning' your life - but here was where we had to step up and live it. A big part of us 'owning' our future was in 'owning' our past. By accepting 100% responsibility for what had happened, we were able to move on with our lives; empowered with having 100% responsibility for our future. Nobody had forced us to transfer our money to a family member who, we knew, had a long track record of dubious dealings. When we heard the alarm bells, we chose to ignore them and stick our head in to the sand and cross our fingers. Just like the children's nursery story 'The Gingerbread Man'; we were the ginger bread man who had agreed to ride on the fox's back across the river, and was subsequently gobbled up. Is the fox to blame for being a fox, or the ginger bread man for not recognising the true nature of a fox? I used to think it was the fox's fault, now I have revised this idea. This collective ownership made us stronger than ever and, with the knowledge that we had brought the problem about ourselves, we felt we also had the power to bring about the necessary actions to augment changes. With this new attitude we were no longer the victims of other people's actions, but took responsibility for our choices, and still do.

We knew that moving our family to the other side of the world and stepping out of the comfort zone required us to take responsibility for our actions. We had always been cocooned (like many of us in the Western world) and lived our lives assuming that if something bad happened then there'd be someone to either fix it or, if not, then someone to blame. Being on the other side of the world, way out of your comfort zone and with the people you love most depending on you, is certainly one way to see what you're made of. You have to adapt and survive, there is no other choice and that is really what human beings have been doing throughout evolution.

Focusing on what we had

One big attitude lesson that we learnt was that we could not continue to focus on the negative aspects of our life. We had to look forward and not back. When we shifted our thinking to focus on all of the good things we had, rather than the bad, we realised how lucky we were. We turned our focus on all of the good things that we had going on with our healthy happy family and, the more we did this, the more we truly valued what we had. Our experience had forced us to turn to the good things and shun the bad and, as a result, we could not help but feel fortunate. All of these amazing things suddenly popped in to our vision that, previously, were just lying dormant in our awareness, being taken for granted. It started out as a forced orientation but, over time, it became a natural way of looking at the world. With this new mind-set we could not help but feel grateful and especially when we would see people who had genuinely been dealt a really tough set of cards, such as handicaps or illnesses. Who on earth were we to feel sorry for ourselves?

To this day, it makes me cringe when I think of how spoilt I had been over the course of my life that I really felt so hard done by, when there are countless people out there in the world who are genuinely struggling with a difficult set of circumstances that life has presented them with. This new way of thinking was such an overwhelming change that my brother wondered if I'd joined some cult or had become religious. This new attitude was nothing that anybody had taught me. It was learnt from my own experience. We will never see our lost money again but we are certainly much richer for the experience and the lessons it taught us. We had to make our own luck and, with hindsight gained a great deal more than we lost.

Which direction to take now?

So we had salvaged our situation to a point; we had escaped from the sinking boat and were now saved and in the life boat. We could now afford a ticket home to the safety and security of our old lives. Now that we had got ourselves back on our feet, we had a new financial challenge on our horizon: a rapidly declining exchange rate. With my being paid in pounds and transferring the money to Australian dollars each month, this declining rate was making a big difference to my salary, and our income. House prices were still going up in Australia and the cost of living with it. This situation was becoming increasingly unsustainable for us and it seemed fate had declared that we were done, and that this was as far as we would be going.

We were at another crossroads and needed to look at the pros and cons of both options. To be honest, at the time the UK option did look appealing; we could go back to our old jobs, our old friends and we would always have some great stories to tell of our great adventure. The exchange rate moves had punished us when bringing money over to Australia but, going the other way, they would be in our favour. The money we had made on the house would be worth more to us in the UK, with this favourable exchange rate.

On the other side of the argument; yes we would have recovered some of our losses, but we felt that we would be going backwards and could not afford the sort of house that we used to live in. My job had changed now and I was not sure what sort of role I would be offered back in the London office, if any. There were other details that we considered, including the fact that we hadn't yet lived in Australia long enough to obtain our Citizenship (dual nationality), but there were two big ones that we couldn't get past.

One: Yes, we were not as wealthy as we used to be but we loved our new life. Seeing the kids grow up living this lifestyle was priceless. We did not have expensive holidays for 14 days of the year anymore, but the 365 days of each year were infinitely better. Two: We would be returning, having failed. Could we go back to all of the things that we wanted to escape in our old lives (the weather, the journey to work, the office environment etc) knowing that was what we would be doing for the rest of our lives? Knowing that we had not crossed the finishing line for our Citizenship would surely compound the bad feeling. If 'what if' was a big factor for us in choosing to come, then it was an even bigger factor in our deciding to stay. We would always be asking; 'what if we had stayed?' We decided to stay.

A new approach
Getting through the previous eighteen months and

renovating our house required a great deal of hard work and frugal living – but that was a salvage operation. There was an end-goal to all of that. Having now decided that we were staying, we needed a new strategy for how we were going to survive and prosper.

The dream was well and truly over and this was real life; but it was good. We had a reasonably large mortgage for our new house, but who doesn't? We had increasingly expensive school fees, now that all three of our kids were at school. There were five people that needed food and clothes. These were all fixed situations that were not going to change, but our income was not fixed but varying wildly and falling fast.

Now our youngest was at school, Angela and I were both able to work full-time and, with the hours available to us without a commute to work; we began to study new financial models that may work for us. With our new found sense of independence and empowerment, we needed to find a mathematical solution to the equation of more money going out than coming in. We looked at our out-goings and compiled an 'essential' and a 'non-essential' list. Anything that was non-essential we got rid of. At this point I should say that many people would consider school fees to be a non-essential, when there is free education available. Common sense would probably say the same thing as our school fees were often as much as our mortgage repayments and, even when we were renovating; many people would have questioned our continuing to keep our kids in private school. Good education has always been important to us and our children were thriving. Throughout everything, we considered that these schools fees were on the 'essential' list (though second hand books and uniforms helped considerably.) We still believe that, although it is not always easy to justify the expense, it is something that is very important to us personally.

We read books on; down-shifting, multiple-streams of income, self-sufficiency, frugal lifestyle strategies, entrepreneurship and many others. As we learnt more we discovered that opportunities were appearing, where we hadn't considered them before. The situation with Angela's business back in the UK was thankfully resolved and we felt we could at last begin to move forward with our new life.

Learning new financial models

In the years that have passed, Angela and I have adopted many of the things that we researched back then. We try to manage our cash-flow quite tightly and keep our regular outgoings to a miniMum by putting things in place that help, such as; using fans instead of air-con, having solar heated water and only owning one car. To lessen the dependency of my salary as a single source of income, we now have additional streams of income such as; part-time jobs, owning a rental home, share-dealing and we have two other businesses that we run together. Our priority has always been our family and so all of these income activities work around our family life - we don't have long commutes to work anymore and so we have more hours available to use productively. Our children have also had to find work for the extras in their lives; such as movies, clothes and mobile phones. This rudimentary understanding of 'earning money in order to spend it' has provided them with a positive attitude towards finances.

A work in progress

Our life is a work in progress, the same as everybody else's. The exchange rate still has a major say in our income and we still work hard in order to get by, just like everybody else. We have started businesses that have failed but we have businesses that continue to do well. We do not have the sort of income that we used to have in the UK, but the lifestyle that we enjoy today more than compensates for that.

We look back at the cossetted life that we lived in the UK and the bullet-proof attitude that we had before we left. Loosening the hold on our money was something we didn't give much thought to, because we felt that nothing could go wrong for us. We were on the crest of a wave. The feeling of buoyancy and excitement that we had when we were starting our new dream life was wonderful - but it wasn't real life. Just as a wedding is a wonderful day - but a marriage is something different, that is built over years together. It's not just one day and a nice dress.

We've recognised the part that we played in losing our money and we've admitted that we were naïve, but I'd hate to think that we could never trust anybody ever again because of one event. Also, I consider that it may well be a part of the natural order of things. Stocks go down as well as up, waves break and people's lives contain good things and bad things - if they didn't life would be pretty dull. A movie about a steady life with everything going well and no bad events to overcome would be pretty dull viewing. In Greek mythology;

'Nemesis' was the goddess of righteous indignation, who punished boasts of 'Hubris' (arrogance before the Gods). Her actions were severe but her task was to maintain equilibrium in human affairs. Maybe Nemesis was just giving us a whack to make sure we were appreciating all of the gifts that we already had. Certainly these events have played their part in teaching us many new and invaluable skills, plus the strength, resourcefulness and resilience required to apply them to our lives.

CHAPTER SUMMARY

Learn from these experiences and use their lessons to make you stronger and more resilient.

Accept that bad things inevitably happen at some point and to prepare a strategy for coping with them next time or avoiding them altogether.

Take the good from difficult situations and feel pride in your ability to deal with them and in coming out of the other side.

Use your new perspective of 'life ownership' to move you forward.

Look at your income streams. If there is too much dependency in one area then use your extra time available to create new additional sources.

14. REINVENTION

'It may be hard for an egg to turn into a bird: it would be a jolly sight harder for it to learn to fly while remaining an egg. We are like eggs at present. And you cannot go on indefinitely being just an ordinary, decent egg. We must be hatched or go bad'
C. S. Lewis

As we discussed in the first part of this book; companies have to continually adapt to changing market conditions. This also applies to the people who work for those companies and we all have to be able to recognise what we offer as a resource, and be proactive in making sure that what we provide stays of value. All of us in the workplace need to keep adapting and evolving our skills, whether we are office based or remote workers.

When I first joined my present company twelve years ago things were very different from today. We were operating in an area that definitely had potential but, as yet, it was still on the way to fruition. We were a bit 'early to the party' and, for the first few years of my being there, we really struggled at times. Since then, however, people's changing use of technology has seen the company go from strength to strength and it is now fulfilling that potential with rapid global expansion.

When I first began working from home eight years ago, it's probably fair to say that I was a reasonable sized fish in a decent sized pond. I was not a big fish in a little pond but even so, I was a middle manager in a decent sized company. I managed a good team, understood our client's needs and how our offering and our business model serviced those needs. When it was first agreed that I continue working for the company, there was a lot of sense in that, as my inherent qualities and experience had value to the company. Today, it's fair to say, that I am far from a big fish in a little pond. I am probably more like a tiny fish in an ocean, whose visibility barely shows up on the company radar at all. But here I am still working from home and still continuing to be a valued employee. In order to achieve that, I have had to keep a close eye on what it is that I am providing to my employer and to keep on adapting, in order to make sure that my contributions stay of value. Just as, how we had to adapt according to the changing circumstances in our personal life, I have also had to adapt to the changing circumstances in my working life. I have had to learn to evolve and, to some extent, to keep on reinventing myself.

However, I would say that this is normal for any employee who has been with a company for twelve years, whether remotely or office based. I do recognise that a twelve year time-span is unusual, by today's standards. Whether I would still be working for the same company after all this time if I was still office based I'm not sure, but with the ability to work remotely on the other side of the world, I consider that I have a very good deal and have striven to maintain this situation over the years. Apparently this is a feeling that is common amongst remote workers as, according to research, there is a culture of 'overcompensation', where employees recognise that they are trusted and are given an opportunity and so feel grateful, empowered and committed to doing a good job, in order to retain that situation. Interestingly, this research goes on to estimate that this 'overcompensation' adds up to an additional twenty four days a year (two days per month) being worked as good will. Add this to the lack of sick days and it's easy to see that the gains are mutually beneficial. The feeling of autonomy is great and definitely inspires me to do a really good job. So, there are definitely on-going benefits to working from home for my employer, but that doesn't change the fact that the person that left the office eight years ago is a very different employee, in terms of a resource, to the one today.

After a few different pitches to a number of potential clients we had some results and these companies had agreed to come aboard with us, on the proviso that we set up an Australian office. This was the perfect start for us as we could now invest in a regional Australian office, with these clients as the foundation for our growth in the region.

I really enjoyed these times where I was getting 'suited and booted' and getting on a plane for meetings. They were exciting experiences and reflected my own feelings of potential towards my own life. It was all new and there were great opportunities for growth and fresh experiences. On the back of these new clients we set up a small office in Sydney and it was manned by a couple of account management guys sent out from the UK. I continued to work remotely from the West coast. All work was still coming out of the hub of our London office and, when I did work for our Australian clients it would come to me from there, via our East coast sales office. One real benefit of having me 'on the ground' here was that I had experience pitching to new clients and so this really helped our getting a foot-hold in the early days. From there I was able to go back to my home office out West and to concentrate on my core job but, another benefit of my being here was that I could potentially move over to Sydney if we started to grow the business and needed production facilities in the region. Having set up and managed a team in London I had the experience to be able to replicate that here, if required. Although I wasn't crazy about the idea of moving to a big city and being office based again, I was not going to discount the possibility of this, as a new challenge always has an appeal. Overtime, we did upscale our operations in the region and started offices in Sydney, Melbourne and Singapore. I never had to relocate to work in any of them but, having me available 'on stand-by', continued to be a 'value-added' reason to retain my services.

As time has gone by, there have been inevitable changes in operations and in personnel. My original boss, who agreed to my coming here, sadly moved on and my colleague with whom I had worked with for so many years (the one I swapped jobs with) has also since moved. With these changes have come inevitable questions asked of me and re-evaluations of my role over the years.

As the years have gone by I have had to continue to assess what I am able to offer my employer and assess its value. This is really no different from an office based employee as we all have to do this throughout the course of our careers, but the difference with a remote worker is that you need to be really aware of these yourself, as there are no visible indicators in your everyday working environment. Taking accountability for your own performance is a 'must have' for anybody that wants to make working from home sustainable. I'm not suggesting that you over-think everything to the point where it creates paranoia about your job, but you do need to have an independent and objective awareness of the value of your role and your performance. Try to step outside of yourself as a person and try and really gauge what you do from a purely resource perspective. Would you continue to employ you? Yes. Great! If not, then why not? Has anything changed in the context and circumstances of your role and, if so, what do you need to do in order to add value in other ways? Can you be nimble enough to make these changes? It's always worth referring back to the 'metrics of your performance' that you hopefully agreed with your boss at the beginning of the arrangement. By reminding yourself how your performance is being gauged, you can get a more accurate feel for what the expectations are from others.

My career path as a remote worker is not as clearly defined as an office based worker. It may be in years to come, when this practice becomes more accepted and conventional but for now it just isn't. My goals and objectives, in a work context, are identified by my boss in an annual review, but my holistic goals and objectives are much broader. Working from home to me is about achieving a work-life balance and so my goals and objectives are about both work and life. At the same time as I have been evolving and reinventing myself as an employee, I have also been evolving and reinventing myself as a person.

I can choose to move to other companies in Australia or in the UK and my company can decide not to employ me anymore. Working from home doesn't suddenly remove all of the usual concerns about your position within a company - if anything it has the potential to heighten your feeling of job insecurity at times. But it can also change your perspective about what it is that you actually do. By assessing yourself, objectively as a resource, it will keep you aware of 'what you bring to the table.'

CHAPTER SUMMARY

Individuals within the workplace need to react to changing conditions, just as companies within the marketplace need to react and adapt to them.

Reinvention is a natural part of growth and evolution, whether office based or a remote worker, and it will ultimately improve your career sustainability prospects.

Accept that there will be inevitable readdressing of the older work-life ratios. To gain an improvement in your personal life you may have to give up something on your professional life.

Retain a focus of the goals you set yourself when you embarked on this. It is about a work-life balance.

DANIEL BOND

15. LIFESTYLE CHANGES

'Boy, those French:
They have a different word for everything'
Steve Martin

Our move has brought about some significant lifestyle changes for us. We still have to do the shopping, cooking, washing and all of the other things that everyday family life requires, but the big difference is the environment that we are doing them in. As with my work; I am still doing the same job, but the big difference is the environment that I'm doing it in. The actual environment that we are living in is so much better and allows us to live the lifestyle that we always dreamed of. However, for the things we have gained in this lifestyle, there are things that we have inevitably missed out on too.

Outdoor life
One big change in our lifestyle is the amount of time we spend outdoors. So much more of life here takes place outdoors and when we look back at photos taken back in the UK we see how much of an indoor existence we led.

Most of our kids play has always been outdoors. It's

important that they still have the option of the modern 'toys' that many of their peer group around the world enjoy (computer games etc), but, over the years, they have chosen to spend most of their time; in the garden on their trampoline swings and tree-house, and out and about; on bikes, skateboards, scooters and surfboards.

Pretty much all of our meals are eaten outside for most of the year and we always make sure, where possible, that we all eat together as a family. Often at weekends we will not eat at home but go to a park for a cook-up, where there are free barbeque facilities.

Most of our socializing generally takes place either in parks or at our home but, either way, it's pretty much always outdoors. The culture in the UK is much more indoors orientated (generally because of the weather). Socializing is generally done at the pub or in the home but it is mostly indoors.

Most movies and concerts that we see are outdoors. We go to the drive-in movies quite often where the kids get in their pyjamas and bundle cushions, blankets and cuddly toys in to the back of the car. We also go to many outdoor movies screenings and concerts. These are generally family orientated events where everybody brings their chairs, picnics and blankets and joins in the fun.

Water
Another big change in our lifestyle is that we spend so much time in the water. Time at the beach or in a swimming pool were very much things that you did on holiday in our old life. This country is built along the

coastlines and water plays a big part in Australian life.

In our new lifestyle a great deal of socializing is done either at the beach or around the pool. We have always loved playing with our kids in the pool and, early on, invented a game called 'Honcho-poncho-loncho' which has been woven in to the fabric of our kids' childhood. The rules are that the kids take it in turns to be thrown in to the air and, while they are airborne, they have to say an agreed word (it's always a made up tongue twister such as; 'Aphabetti-spaghetti on the jetty' or something along those lines). They get a point if they manage to say the whole phrase before going under the water. There is a different word for each round and the word for the final round is always 'Honcho-poncho-loncho'. The game lasts for as long as our arms can keep throwing kids in to the air; so it has become an increasingly shorter game as the years have gone by and the kids have grown bigger. Soon they will be throwing us.

I love it that our kids childhood memories will include playing Honcho-poncho-loncho in a swimming pool on a hot day, rather than just watching TV, because it's raining outside and Dad had to work again at the weekend.

Weather
When I was growing up in England, I never thought about the weather. I was out playing all of the time and sometimes I would come inside and my Mum would point out that I was soaking wet and covered in mud, and other times she would point out that I was soaking wet and covered in sweat. I was oblivious to any of this

until she pointed it out. This blissful ignorance was, in part; because I was a kid and too busy playing and, in part; because these things had not been switched on in my awareness.

Since those days, progress has brought about so much more information, presented us with more opportunities and opened up so many windows in to other worlds. TV shows from around the world have brought about an awareness of how people live in other countries. Foreign travel has allowed us to experience different cultures, languages and different climates. Globalisation has brought about international trade and provided us with a variety of products from all around the world.

In the context of British weather, we have opened up 'Pandora's Box'. We have seen how people spend their wonderful sunny summer days in American movies. We love spending a fortnight sunbathing in Continental Europe each year for our holidays. We buy light-weight summer clothing and barbeques each year in preparation for that long hot summer that we see on the TV adverts.

The point I am getting to here, is that the UK has not moved, and is not suddenly getting temperate weather conditions – it always has. Nobody ever expected to have barbeques or swimming pools in the past but we do now; and we are upset when the rain comes and spoils it. We have seen how others live and we want it for ourselves. The British weather has always been inclement; we just didn't have much else to compare it to. I put my hand up and say that I am one of those who had become dissatisfied with British weather. I had experienced better weather in other countries and I liked it.

The weather that we enjoy in our new lifestyle is wonderful. We have nine months of clear skies and, what is best described as, a Mediterranean climate. We have three months of cool temperatures when it rains and fills the damns and lakes back up. The heat is dry and not humid and the weather patterns are predictable - if it's sunny in the morning, it'll be sunny all day. The good weather also has a hand in creating a laid back, positive attitude. People don't feel inclined to complain so much; and those routine activities that we mentioned previously (washing, shopping etc) just don't seem as bad when you're doing them under a blue sky.

What we have given up to enjoy this lifestyle
The lifestyle that we enjoy today is exactly the sort of thing that we imagined all those years ago, and so we consider ourselves to be very fortunate. However, this hasn't come without consequence and there are many things that this lifestyle does not feature.

We have no immediate family near us and, as we live so far away it is expensive for us to travel back and for our friends and relatives to come and visit us. As a consequence; our kids have missed out on having an extended family involved in their lives and, the more time goes by, the older and more distant these relatives become.

As well as the kids missing out on these family connections, Angela and I have missed our families and friends. These personal relationships are not only important in day to day life but they are also a large part of our own personal histories. As you get older it becomes harder to make new friends and people often rely more heavily on the relationships that they established earlier on in their lives. When you relocate you are forced to create new relationships and this requires having to get out of your comfort zone to do so. It's often only when you are forced to establish new relationships that you realise how much you valued your old ones.

As well as your personal history vanishing, to some extent; your personal identity is also something of the past. As we have mentioned in the book already; a readdressing of your work-life balance does often mean something of a revaluation of your professional identity. We may not always like being judged and pigeon-holed so much by what we do, but it can also be something of a comfort. Many of us work very hard to establish a good career for ourselves and the perception of our status and recognition of our achievements is something that feels good. Working from home is in many ways a blank sheet of paper and your identity will be revaluated and your past achievements will not be known or recognised.

We have been fortunate that I have been able to continue to work remotely for this amount of time. However in that time-frame, many of my peer group have progressed with their careers, whereas mine has very much plateaued, and my salary scale with it. If you are looking to make a move to working from home then you have to recognise that it is unlikely your career will advance at the same pace as your office based peers. This may change in the future but for now it is something that you have to factor in as part of the deal.

Probably the most significant thing that we have missed out on is the feeling of security. This feeling is made up of a combination of familiar things and people. When we have experienced problems we have had none of our old personal network or familiar routines to help us through them, but as we said earlier; you cannot ask for change, and not expect change.

CHAPTER SUMMARY

The lifestyle that we enjoy today is almost exactly what we pictured for ourselves all those years ago.

Picture the lifestyle you want for yourself. What does it consist of?

For all of the things you gain there will be an inevitable amount of things that you miss out on.

Look at the things you may potentially miss out on and consider ways that you could prepare for these, or avoid them altogether (for example; would your parents consider relocating with you?)

16. THE BEST OF BOTH WORLDS

'Live life in a Holiday mood'
JB Priestly

I would say one of the great things about working from home is the feeling of having the best of both worlds. You have the opportunity to pursue your lifestyle ambitions while still being able to continue with your career. Also, if you have relocated to a new environment then you are able to experience this while still being able to return to your previous office based environment on occasion too.

Although technology allows me to fulfil my working commitments from a completely remote location, I still go back to the UK about once a year. This is invaluable as it enables me to maintain good personal relationships with my work colleagues and to meet new co-workers that I may have been working closely with for some time, but have not actually met in person yet. It is also an opportunity to put my laptop in for a 'pit-stop' with the technical support department who can make sure that my software is up to date and that my hard-ware is still in good working order. The frequency of my trips has varied over the years, but I have generally found that one annual trip works well for me.

These trips back are a very important part of the whole package of my working from home. My ability to work remotely for the vast majority of the year is very much aided by the short time spent in the office collaborating on projects and fostering good relationships each year. This is of value to me and also to my employer; as it improves the overall working relationships and ultimately the output of the work.

Providing a context

I would probably say the biggest benefit of these trips back for me, is that they provide me with an invaluable context to my working and personal life. It is a part of the human-condition to stop noticing the everyday things around us and, as a consequence, to stop appreciating them. I really do appreciate the fortunate working situation that I have, but I am only human and over the years have come to think of it as 'normal' and to take it for granted. These trips back really help me to refresh that appreciation and to motivate me in continuing to work hard to maintain it. It really doesn't take long; after just one day commuting in to the office I am longing for my two second office commute at home and am so grateful for the lifestyle that I have. As I said at the start of this book, I have written this to me ten years ago and I know he's still out there (or rather people who still share that situation) because I see him or her on these trips back every time I get on the commuter train.

When I'm back I experience; the train delays and

cancellations; the blanket of grey cloud that hangs over peoples' day; the intensity of the high-demand treadmill that so many people struggle to maintain each day and the impolite, stressed out attitude that their anxiety often manifests itself into. I experience the sterile and soul-less silence of office life, that seems to make each working day last forever. Basically, I am fortunate that I get to revisit all of my original motivations for my starting out on this journey in the first place.

I know I paint a bleak picture of the working day but there are also many things that I do miss and it is a great thing for me to have the opportunity to go back so that I can do these things as well. When I'm back I love to spend time with my family, to meet up with old friends and to do all of the little things that I miss being able to do on a regular basis.

I also like the sense of 'duality' in my experience of going back. I have to take both passports with me and so I enter the UK as a British Citizen and then return home as an Australian Citizen. I like the feeling that I am able to experience both countries and appreciate them both, for different reasons. One of the things that suits me about working from home is that I don't feel 'locked in' to one place or another. These trips back really make me feel like I have the 'best of both worlds'. I love my new surroundings but am glad to still be working in my chosen career and really like still being a part of that world. The work challenges me and I am able to feel a part of the modern, technical and innovative world, while still being able to enjoy the simple pleasures that my new environment provides me with.

One particular occasion that I remember really experiencing the feeling of having the best of both worlds was when I had just returned from a trip back to London office a few years ago. Each year, my son Michael and I go camping on an annual 'Fathers and sons weekend' in the bush, with a small group of other Dads and sons. It was really important to both me and my son that I manage to make the trip and so I booked my flights to ensure that I would be back in time, and got home the night before we left. On that occasion I had only been in the UK office for two days and, suffice to say, I was exhausted and thoroughly jet-lagged.

On the Saturday night Michael awoke in pain in the middle of the night. He was having cramps in his legs, probably brought about by the cold of the night and so we went out to the camp fire to warm up. We sat by the fire together under the Southern Cross and a beautifully clear night sky. I thought how lucky I was that, a few hours ago, I was in a beautiful English pub having a pint with my brother and here I was under a blanket of stars on the other side of the planet with my little boy.

Overall I would say that, to me, 'going back' is an essential ingredient in helping me to 'go forward'. It provides me with; perspective, appreciation, context, motivation and helps to keep me on track. It's like reviewing a brief or running through blue-prints in order to make sure that I'm still building that dream that I set out to build. Going back is great but, without a doubt, the best part of all is coming home again. Being greeted at the airport by my family with a hand-made welcome home card is definitely always the best bit.

The difference between overseas working from home and emigration

This feeling of 'having the best of both worlds' is great on the occasions when I do get to spend time experiencing both worlds, but how does it play out for the rest of the time?

If you are working remotely overseas in a foreign country; what's the difference between working from home and emigrating? In practical, day to day terms; nothing much; but I would say the main difference is in attitude. We always said we were coming for two years and have always approached it as an 'overseas posting' or 'secondment'. We don't know if we'll be here forever but, right now, it is a good place for us to be. Earlier on in the book we looked at combining the working from home options available and, for us; we can potentially move to a new location within Australia, or we could move back to the UK and continue working from home. Having these options available to my wife and I has a positive effect on our attitude and is one of the aspects that we really like about my working from home.

As we said earlier; things that are familiar can easily become, well... familiar. How many of us take a tourist excursion around our home town? People will travel to other countries to look around their cities and explore their history and culture, but will seldom get on a tourist bus and discover all about the city they live in. We just don't see our everyday environment in the same way. When your mind-set determines that you *live* somewhere, then your attitude and actions are entirely different to the mind-set of *visiting*. When moving to a new environment this is something you come to recognise.

Being aware of this, we try to maintain that 'visiting' mind-set whenever we can. When we go back to London we appreciate, like never before, the history and the architecture available. Likewise when we come back to Australia we try to appreciate the beaches and the blue skies like we are on holiday here. It's not always easy as we humans and, by nature, take note of the new things in our experience and disregard or just accept the everyday familiar things - it's probably a part of a hard-coded survival instinct. However, we have found that assuming the attitude that we don't know how long we'll be here definitely helps to keep that freshness and keeps us from taking things too much for granted. This may not work for everybody, as other people find comfort in familiar things and may be more 'homely' people by nature. I think Angela and I probably have nomadic tendencies in us and are both equally stimulated by the idea of experiencing new places. Remote overseas working and the inherent attitude that it brings, luckily seems to suits us.

CHAPTER SUMMARY

Working from home enables you to experience the feeling of having best of both worlds, both with your personal and professional life, and also in your geography.

Going back to your former location helps provide a valuable context.

The inherent attitudes between *visiting* somewhere and *living* somewhere are very different.

17. HAVE WE ACHIEVED WHAT WE SET OUT TO?

'A mind that is stretched by a new experience
can never go back to its old dimensions'
Oliver Wendell Holmes, Jr

For me, it's a solid yes. We have absolutely achieved what we set out to. It hasn't gone to plan but perhaps 'throwing away the plan' was actually the point.

My two primary motivations were 'more family time' and 'the opportunity to experience new things' and these were intrinsically linked. If I had simply wanted to gain more family time then I could have achieved this by moving closer to the office. Likewise, if I had just wanted the opportunity to experience new things then I could have moved overseas and spent all my time scuba-diving, mountain climbing and countless other new experiences. For me, the real magic has been in the combination of both of these; in having the time to experience new things *together* with my family.

I have written about just a few stories of some of the experiences that we've shared together. They are all a part of the journey that we have travelled as a family, and we probably have enough stories to fill ten books. We have had big adventures and countless little ones. The thing that has bound our personal history together so tightly is the little ones. The big adventures are like the bricks and all of the countless small events and experiences are the mortar cement that makes it solid.

I love experiencing the big stuff with my family but best of all I love being around to do the small stuff. For me, the secret ingredient in all of this is time. It's said to be the most valued commodity of all and one that even the wealthiest of men cannot buy more of. Our daughters both remember their old school lives in the UK, and they have always said that they love it that one of us has always been home after school, rather than them having to go off to day-care until we return home from work.

There are so many seemingly small activities that I've been able to share over the last eight years that I would never had had time for in my old life. Had I always been able to do these little things with my kids then I may not have appreciated the last eight years so much but, having had the experience of my old life to compare it to, it's something I do truly value.

When it isn't new anymore

All of the experiences that I described in the first half of this book were very exciting for us. They were all new and were exactly what we were looking for: *new* experiences. Eight years on, those things are no longer new to us. Kangaroos, scorching sun, beautiful beaches; these have now become normal for us. This lifestyle is now one that Angela and I have adapted to and we don't think about the differences very often any more. Our kids don't really have a comparison and, for them, it is normal. So, what happens when the things that were new become accepted and familiar? Do they lose their appeal? We're all familiar with the phrase the 'honeymoon period' and really this applies to our experience here. To extend the metaphor; we had a great honeymoon period but that has developed in to a wonderful marriage that has had its ups and downs, but has been made all the better for them. The new things have lost their shine, but not their appeal.

We have established our own traditions, some of which are very different from the ones that we used to have in the UK, but they are an integral part of our family life. Christmas, for example, is hot in Australia and you'd think it wouldn't quite be the same as the winter ones that we grew up with, but I love our Australian Christmases and we're really used to them now. It isn't clearly better or clearly worse; it's just different in so many ways that it's not really comparable. Christmas here is just a part of summer, where the weather is hot, everybody is at the beach or in the pool, there are great outdoor events on and many people are going away on their holiday. Plus, we also host a 'Christmas in July' each year for about twenty of our closest friends. It's a great day with everybody contributing and even the big man makes an appearance with a little gift, for all those not on the naughty list.

Changing motivations
Our objectives for coming here were based on the needs of Angela and myself. We came here to address our own needs; as adults and as parents. Sure, we were

thinking of our kids' upbringing but it was our decision and not theirs. Our lifestyle choices were made for a young family and while sunshine, simplicity and consistency are important for young kids, for older kids and young adults these things may not be so important. Their needs change as they get older and become more independent. The needs of a collective of five people gradually evolve in to the needs of five unique individuals. Now, at the time of writing; Florence is eighteen, Alice is fourteen and Michael is nine.

We all know how time seems to fly by at times in our life, and never more so than when our kids get older. Eight years is about one fifth of my life so far. It's not a huge slice of my life-span so far, but in the context of a child's life, it is a huge amount of time. So many changes occur within that time-frame in childhood that it sometimes seems as though somebody is pushing the fast-forward button in your own life.

Luckily for us, our children are all very contented and we have a great relationship as a family. Angela has a great saying, she says; 'Raising children is like growing your own friends'. I love that and it really is a great representation of the sort of person she is and why she is loved and admired by so many. I am so proud of my family and I couldn't be happier with the wonderful friends that Angela and I are growing. They really are our best friends and we are very proud of them all.

When our eldest daughter Florence turned eighteen we had an assessment together of where we were; based on her needs, now and in the future. After considering all aspects, we all decided that this was still the best place for her as she has great friends, she can afford to go to University here and there are much better career prospects for her at present. She is very happy with her life and we are glad that we have played our part in helping to provide her with the opportunities that she has today. This was the most recent occasion where we assessed where we were based on everybody's needs, and we will do it again when we need to. She is now doing really well at University and has also taken a trip back the UK on her own (funded by her part time jobs). She was happy to be able to go back and tap in to the English part of her but was even more happy to return home to her family and friends - she is also enjoying the best of both worlds now in the way that I do when I go back to the UK office.

So, we have created a new 'norm' and this may become something that we may decide to move on from at some point in the future. Angela and I wanted to experience 'different' - well it may be that our kids want to experience 'different' when they're older too. If they do, then they will have the opportunity to do so (as they have dual nationality) and they will have our blessing, and full encouragement to live their lives to the fullest and to take advantage of all life's opportunities (although they know us well enough to know that we may well arrive on their doorstep anytime, wherever that doorstep might be.)

In summary, to answer the question; have we achieved what we set out to achieve? Yes. We could never have guessed what was in store for us and it has certainly been a very different reality to the one that we dreamed about, but it has provided us with exactly what we needed, and so much more besides.

CHAPTER SUMMARY

Your overall achievement can be determined by measuring your reality against the objectives you set yourself before making your change in lifestyle.

If this is to be a sustainable option for you then you will need to consider that your objectives may change as time goes by and that a revaluation of your needs may be required from time to time.

Things are very exciting when they are new, but will they still appeal to you in the same way when they are not new anymore?

Over time you will inevitably create a new 'norm.' Will this still satisfy your needs in the same way?

SAME JOB NEW LIFE

18. WHERE TO FROM HERE?

**'Life can only be understood backwards;
but it must be lived forwards'**
Soren Kierkegaard

These years in Australia have been a rare exception in my life where I have been able to isolate a specific time-frame and analyse the events that have taken place and consider all that we have learnt. This opportunity for retrospection has been healthy in so many ways and has helped us to evaluate some of the experiences and to apply what we have learnt in new and positive ways.

One pattern that we have seen repeated throughout our experience in all of this is that the 'old sayings' keep coming back to us and proving that they were right all along. There is an enormous archive of old sayings that is stored somewhere in in the library of the 'collective unconscious.' We are all told them throughout the course of our lives, and they are generally given in the form of advice for things that are yet to come. Sage advice on things that we are yet to experience with the aim of preparing us for when they do. When I think back over this eight year period, I've actually found it has happened the other way for us: We have experienced something that has perhaps taken months or years and has perhaps been painful or difficult to fully understand and then, we are reminded of some of 'old saying,' that we've always known, and it actually captures exactly that we have been through, and encapsulates it in a single sentence.

This is very much true with the saying *'It's not about the destination, it's about the journey'*. We've all heard this one but, if there was a single sentence that encapsulates everything that we have been through and our feelings towards our life right now, it is this. We have spent years learning this (and I have spent a whole book trying to articulate it) and there it was all along; the lesson was there already in a single sentence - but without the experience, it doesn't have the same resonance or power.

So, if I had to identify where we are now and where are heading, I would simply say that we are somewhere on our journey. We still have goals that we want to achieve and we have a general direction that we want to head in, but we don't have such a strong determination and focus on the 'destination' anymore. We began this journey looking for a destination that would provide a reward for all of our hard work and sacrifice. We were looking for a life package; all boxed up and ready to go. We have learnt that it just doesn't work like that and that the 'destination' is actually found embedded *within* the 'journey'. The life that we were seeking has been found on the journey, and that the 'destination' was only ever a figment of our imagination. This journey has created an amazing lifestyle for us and hopefully it will continue for a long time to come, but I don't know if we'll ever reach a destination as such. We could relocate somewhere else and continue working from home, but we are currently still happy with our present location.

I think if you had to translate what the 'destination' is in the modern working culture, it would perhaps be retirement. There is a famous psychology principle of 'delayed gratification' which measures how children who can demonstrate the ability to resist the temptation for an immediate reward and wait for a later reward, will potentially go on to achieve more in their adult lives. This principle is very important in the development and maturity of individuals and how they contribute to the society that we all live in, however in the context of what we are looking at here; there is perhaps a case to suggest that we may be taking the concept of 'deferred gratification' too far. If we are denying ourselves too many of the good things (family time, happiness, personal reward etc) until such a time that we may be too old to really enjoy them; then is this wise? If there are other ways that allow us to balance some of the reward *now* while still working towards and investing our time and efforts in achieving further rewards *in the future*, then shouldn't we explore these options? I really think that working from home has the potential to offer us a good balance with work-life and also reward now/reward later.

The bigger journey
For me, working from home has been a part of bigger journey; one where I have discovered the importance of self-reliance and the joy of independence. My attitude

in my old office based life was one of *entitlement*; where I believed I had the right to good life, just so long as I kept on working hard and doing all of the things that were expected of me. Like that of a child to their parent; if I did what I was told then my employer would always look after me. I think that attitude is probably something that has been carried over from previous generations and I would suggest that, in today's changing world, it may not be entirely relevant. The world and our workplaces are changing at such a rate of knots that we need to be able to adapt our thinking to match these changes and to advance our own opportunities.

Another one of those familiar phrases that we've discovered to be true is; *'You work to live, not live to work.'* Again, another old favourite that we're all familiar with but this never had the same level of significance to me as it does now. Now I understand it. The opportunity to work remotely has enabled me to find a work-life balance that I am happy with. My working has been there to finance and facilitate my lifestyle; I have been working to live. In my old life 'who I was' was defined by my job title and I had to dedicate so many hours to working and the logistics of working (eg; travelling etc), that I had very little time for anything else, or to learn to be anybody else; I was living to work.

At some time in the future, my employer and I will part ways. I am no hurry to bring this about but it is inevitable, just as it would be if I were office based. I will always be grateful to my company for allowing me the opportunity to work remotely. I have thoroughly enjoyed the experience but, more than that, it has enabled me to learn new ways of living (and to make a living) that is not wholly derived from a single source of a salary. My salary is a very welcome part of a number of different streams of income, rather than the single one that we are wholly dependent upon. As I have said before, financially we are not rich. This is not one of those books that is written retrospectively by a 'guru', looking back on the various events and hard-times that were endured in order to get the writer to the comfortable position that they enjoy today. This one is not like that. This is it folks. There is no agenda to further the advance of working from home or a war cry for everybody to 'down-tools' and do the same as me. As I have said throughout this book; I do not believe that working from home will be the right thing for everybody, nor do I realistically see a time in the very near future where working from home becomes the norm. If, however, it is the right thing for you at this point in your life then I sincerely hope that this book has helped to serve as an inspiration and will help to guide you on your own journey.

As for us; we will certainly never regret taking the path less travelled. By gaining the priceless gift of time and sharing in the many adventures and experiences with our family, we will always be glad we came. We are sometimes asked the question, 'Would we ever go back?' Our answer is simple: 'No. We will go forward; wherever that may be.'

CHAPTER SUMMARY

My attitude in my old office based life was one of entitlement. I have now learnt the importance of self-reliance and the joy of freedom.

'It is about the journey; not the destination.'

'You work to live, not live to work.'

The experience of working from home enables us the opportunity to have a fuller life, and to learn so much more than simply replicating what we've always done, but from another location.

ABOUT THE AUTHOR

Daniel Bond lives and works in Western Australia, with his wife and three children

www.ingramcontent.com/pod-product-compliance
Lightning Source LLC
Chambersburg PA
CBHW071346290326
41933CB00041B/2764